Disorders of Human Learning, Behavior, and Communication

Ronald L. Taylor and Les Sternberg
Series Editors

Don C. Van Dyke David J. Lang
Frances Heide Susan van Duyne
M. Joan Soucek
Editors

Clinical Perspectives in the Management of Down Syndrome

Springer-Verlag
New York Berlin Heidelberg
London Paris Tokyo Hong Kong

Senior Editors: Don C. Van Dyke, Department of Pediatrics, The University of Iowa Hospitals and Clinics, Iowa City, IA 52242, U.S.A.
David J. Lang, Children's Hospital of Orange County, Orange, CA 92668, U.S.A.
Frances Heide, San Gabriel Pomona Regional Center, West Covina, CA 91790, U.S.A.

Associate Editors: Susan van Duyne, Chicago, IL 60181, U.S.A.
M. Joan Soucek, Division of Developmental Disabilities, The University of Iowa Hospitals and Clinics, Iowa City, IA 52242, U.S.A.

Series Editors: Ronald L. Taylor and Les Sternberg, Exceptional Student Education, Florida Atlantic University, Boca Raton, FL 33431-0991, U.S.A.

Library of Congress Cataloging–in–Publication Data
Clinical perspectives in the management of Down syndrome/Don C. Van Dyke ... [et al.], editors.
p. cm.—(Disorders of human learning, behavior, and communication)
Bibliography: p.
Includes index.
$60.00 (est.)
1. Down's syndrome. I. Van Dyke, Don C. II. Series.
[DNLM: 1, Down's Syndrome. WS 107 C641]
RJ506.D68C55 1989
618.92'858842—dc20
DNLM/DLC 89-6195

Printed on acid free paper.

Softcover reprint of the hardcover 1st edition 1990

Typeset by Thomson Press (India) Limited, New Delhi, India.

9 8 7 6 5 4 3 2 1

ISBN-13: 978-1-4613-9646-8 e-ISBN-13: 978-1-4613-9644-4
DOI: 10.1007/978-1-4613-9644-4

Foreword

The management of and attitudes toward children and adults with Down syndrome have undergone considerable changes in the course of the condition's long history (Zellweger, 1977, 1981, Zellweger & Patil, 1987). J.E.D. Esquirol (1838) and E. Séguin (1846) were probably the first physicians to witness the condition without using currently accepted diagnostic designations. Séguin coined the terms *furfuraceus* or *lowland cretinism* in contradistinction to the goiterous cretinism endemic at that time in the Swiss Alps. Esquirol, as well as Séguin, had a positive attitude toward persons who were mentally ill or mentally subnormal. Esquirol pioneered a more humane treatment in mental institutions and Séguin created the first homes in France, and later in the United States, aimed at educating persons who were mentally subnormal. The term *mongolian idiocy* was coined by J.H.L. Down in England (1866). The term is misleading in several respects: (1) Down identified the epicanthic folds seen in many children with Down syndrome with the additional skin fold in the upper lid occurring particularly in people of Oriental (Mongolian) descent; and (2) Down also erred by assuming that Down syndrome represented regression to an ethnic variant of lower cultural standing. Such an interpretation might have been understandable at a time when the myth of Anglo-Saxon superiority was widely accepted by the British. Charles Darwin's then highly acclaimed theory of origin of the species may have contributed to such a concept. In spite of this racial chauvinism, Down described the "mongoloid" phenotype in a masterly and unsurpassed fashion, yet his publication shows a therapeutic nihilism, which was shared by other authors who wrote about this syndrome in the second half of the 19th century. Terms like *mongolian idiocy, mongolian imbecility* and *Kalmuc idiocy* (Fraser & Mitchell, 1876) vividly illustrate a negative attitude toward Down syndrome that prevailed well into the first half of the 20th century. Many physicians practicing in those days refused to treat infants with Down syndrome, did not allow the parents to even see their newborn child if it had Down syndrome, and hastened to entomb the child in an institution for the severely handicapped; an action for which many parents never forgave their doctor. Developmental potentials of the children—now well recognized—were fully overlooked.

The discovery of a chromosomal anomaly as the cause of Down syndrome, described in spring 1959 by Lejeune, Gautier, and Turpin and by Jacob, Baikie, Court-Brown, and Strong aroused interest, intense research, and was to precipitate a flood of publications. Results of the various research endeavors led to two different approaches with respect to this syndrome: (1) prenatal diagnosis of Down syndrome, and (2) increased postnatal therapy for persons having this syndrome.

In the late 1960s and early 1970s the combination of amniocentesis and chromosome analysis of the amniotic fluid cells led to a new science: prenatal cytogenetics. It became possible to diagnose the chromosomal anomaly in early pregnancy. With this new technology we are now able to offer parents information to help them decide whether to continue or to terminate the pregnancy. If the parents choose to continue the pregnancy, education about caring for an infant with Down syndrome can better prepare the family to meet their infant's needs.

Medical and educational attitudes toward the child with Down syndrome have made enormous progress in the last 25 years, progress that began in the early 1960s when President John F. Kennedy established a national commission for mental retardation. This commission, after many sessions, concluded that any child with mental retardation has the right to be educated to reach his or her potential. The commission's proposal was legalized in 1975 by Public Law, which stipulates that a free and appropriate public education must be available to every child, regardless of intellectual or physical disability. Associations of parents of children with Down syndrome were formed to safeguard the rights of their children in accordance with the mandate of PL 94–142.

Beginning in the early 1970s, beneficial results of early intervention began to appear in the medical and psychological literature. It has become quite clear that astounding results can be obtained by joint efforts of a team of specialists well versed in different aspects of the complex needs of the child with Down syndrome.

This book, *Clinical Perspectives in the Management of Down Syndrome*, is a splendid example of what such joint efforts can achieve. Edited by two pediatricians, a nurse, a psychologist, and an administrator, it contains contributions from more than 20 specialists. The multiple problems that children with Down syndrome present are lucidly and competently dealt with by specialists of cardiology, ophthalmology, otolaryngology, endocrinology, hematology-oncology, dentistry, orthopedics, speech pathology, psychology, and rehabilitation. In addition, a parent of a child with Down syndrome discusses the initial anguish upon learning the medical diagnosis, and the later joy parents experience with each step in the child's growth and development.

References

Down, J.H.L. (1866). Observations on an ethnic classification of idiots. *Clinical Lectures and Reports, London Hospital, 3*, 259–262.

Esquirol, J.E.D. (1838). Des maladies mentales considerées sons les rapports médicanx, hygiéniques et médicanx-légals, Paris, Baillèrls.

Fraser, M.B., & Mitchell, A. (1876). 'Kalmuc idiocy.' *Journal of Mental Science, 22*, 169–179.

Jacobs, P.A., Baikie, A.G., Court-Brown, W.M., & Strong, J.A. (1959). The somatic chromosomes in Mongolism. *Lancet, 1*, 710–711.

Lejeune, J., Gautier, M. & Turpin, R. (1959). Études des chromosomes somatiques de neuf enfants *mongoliens, C.R. Acad Sci (Paris), 248*, 1721–1722.

Séguin, E. (1846). *Idiocy: Its treatment by the physiological mthod.* New York: W. Wood, Publisher.

Zellweger, H. (1977) Down Syndrome. *Handbook of Clinical Neurology, 31*, 368–469.

Zellweger, H. (1981). The story of Down's syndrome which preceded Langdon Down, *Down Syndrome, 4:1*, 1–2.

Zellweger, H. & Patil, S.R. (1987). Down syndrome. *Handbook of Clinical Neurology, 50:1*, 519–538.

Hans U. Zellweger

Preface

The strength of this book lies in the contributions of more than 20 authors representing numerous disciplines in the fields of medicine, psychology, dentistry, nursing, and rehabilitation. The challenge lay in the blending of the many disciplines to address multiple areas of interest in the clinical management of persons having Down syndrome. In this volume, clinical research areas are addressed in Part I (Chapters 1–13). Although all aspects of the vast body of knowledge about Down syndrome cannot be dealt with in a single book, an effort has been made here to cover some key issues with some of those present in Part II of this book (Chapters 14–19).

The strength of presentation comes from the clinical expertise of the contributors; an extensive literature review; the individual, grant-funded research of many of the investigators; and an analysis of a data base compiled from the case histories of a large number of individuals with Down syndrome, who were seen at Los Angeles Children's Hospital and the Down Syndrome Program at the City of Hope National Medical Center.

The text will prove useful for persons who need both practical and theoretical information about Down syndrome, whether they be parents or professional staff such as therapists, physicians, nurses, or educators. We feel this book provides new perspectives on a variety of management issues and will continue to prove useful to all individuals involved in meeting the needs of the individual with Down syndrome.

Don C. Van Dyke
David J. Lang

Preface

Acknowledgments

We wish to acknowledge the many individuals who have graciously and without remuneration contributed their expertise to the development of this book. We are especially indebted to the professional staff of the Divisions of Developmental Disabilities and Medical Genetics, of the Department of Pediatrics, The University of Iowa Hospitals and Clinics, for their expertise and their patience in the preparation and refinement of this manuscript. In particular, we thank Janice L. Held (The University of Iowa) and Rachel Notarte (USC-Irvine) for technical assistance, Dr. Marie Klugman (Biostatistical Center) and Mr. John Wadsworth (University Hospital School) at the University of Iowa, and Dr. L. Robert Hill at the City of Hope, National Medical Center, for statistical and data support in accumulating and analyzing the computerized data. In addition, our thanks to Mr. Richard T. Huber at the University of Iowa for graphic art.

Special thanks are extended to Dr. Hans Zellweger for his "Foreword," to Dr. Louise R. Greenswag for her encouragement and expertise, to Ms. Susan S. Eberly, Division of Developmental Disabilities, for her editorial expertise, and to the excellent staff of Springer-Verlag Publishers.

We thank the parents and professional group of the City of Hope and the Los Angeles chapter of the National Down Syndrome Congress. Finally, and most important, we are deeply indebted to the individuals with Down syndrome and to their families who allowed us to access their thoughts and ideas, and who served as "splendid examples in our joint efforts" to bring this book to press.

Don C. Van Dyke

Contents

Contributors

Marion Taylor Baer, Ph.D., R.D., University Affiliated Program, Center for Child Development and Developmental Disorders, Los Angeles Children's Hospital, Los Angeles, CA, U.S.A.

Warren S. Brown, Ph.D., Graduate School of Psychology, Fuller Theological Seminary, Pasadena, CA, U.S.A.

Robert W. Borghi, Ph.D., CCC-Sp, Speech and Language Pathology, The City of Hope National Medical Center, Duarte, CA, U.S.A.

Hyejung Chang, M.S. Biostatistical Center, The University of Iowa, Iowa City, IA, U.S.A.

Walter M. Fierson, M.D., F.A.A.O., F.A.A.P., Pediatric Ophthalmology, Los Angeles Children's Hospital/University of Southern California, Los Angeles, CA, U.S.A.

Cheryl A. Gahagen, M.S., R.P.T., Department of Rehabilitation, The City of Hope National Medical Center, Duarte, CA, U.S.A.

L. Stephen Gordon, M.D., Pediatric Cardiology, Cedar-Sinai Medical Center, University of Southern California, Los Angeles, CA, U.S.A.

Heather Gumm, M.A., R.D., Pediatric Nutrition, The City of Hope National Medical Center, Duarte, CA, U.S.A.

Frances Heide, M.S., R.N., San Gabriel/Pomona Regional Center, West Covina, CA, U.S.A.

William G. Hemenway, M.D., Otolaryngology, Portland, OR, U.S.A.

Marty Novak Hoffman, M.A. O.T.R., Department of Rehabilitation, The City of Hope National Medical Center, Duarte, CA, U.S.A.

Robert A. Krance, M.D. Pediatric Hematology/Oncology, The Children's Hospital of Orange County Orange County, CA, U.S.A.

David J. Lang, M.D., Pediatrician-in-Chief, Children's Hospital of Orange County, Orange, CA, U.S.A.

Oariona Lowe, D.D.S., M.S., Department of Pediatric Dentistry, University of California, Los Angeles, Los Angeles, CA, U.S.A.

Laura F. Meyers, Ph.D., Research Linguist, Department of Linguistics, University of California, Los Angeles, Los Angeles, CA, U.S.A.

John D. Miller, M.D., Pediatric Endocrinology, Department of Pediatrics, University of California, Irvine, Irvine, CA, U.S.A.

Toni Monson, President, Down Syndrome Parents and Professional Group, LaVerne, CA, U.S.A.

Linda Lusardi Peterson, B.S., O.T.R., Casa Colina Career Developmental Center, LaVerne, CA, U.S.A.

Maurice E. Popejoy, M.A., CCC-A, Communication Disorders Department, Rancho Los Amigos Medical Center, Downey, CA, U.S.A.

Stacy L. Schantz, Ph.D., Department of Neuropsychology, Neuropsychiatric Institute, University of California, Los Angeles, Los Angeles, CA, U.S.A.

Susan van Duyne, Ed.D., Child Psychology, Chicago, IL, U.S.A.

Don C. Van Dyke, M.D., Division of Development Disabilities, Department of Pediatrics, The University of Iowa Hospitals and Clinics, Iowa City, IA, U.S.A.

Jan Waldron, B.S., R.D., Pediatric Nutrition, Ventura County Medical Center, Ventura, CA, U.S.A.

Hans U. Zellweger, M.D., Division of Medical Genetics, Department of Pediatrics, The University of Iowa Hospitals and Clinics, Iowa City, IA, U.S.A.

Ruth Zemke, Ph.D., O.T.R., Department of Occupational Therapy, University of Southern California, Los Angeles, CA, U.S.A.

Introduction

This book is based in large part on the clinical research done during the development and review of an interdisciplinary program for persons with Down syndrome. This program was open to all individuals with Down syndrome with most participants residing in the Los Angeles, California, area. The program reviewed was modeled after other multidisciplinary programs, with a number of major components coming from the Down Syndrome Program at The University of Maryland developed by Dr. David J. Lang.

One-hundred-ninety individuals aged 2 months to 19 years were involved in this program over the 18-month period in which data was collected (1984–1986). The patient population included a relatively even distribution of females (52%) and males (48%) and the racial distribution showed a predominance of Caucasians and Hispanics. All socioeconomic classes were represented. The distribution of ages was skewed toward the population of 4 years of age and younger. The demographics of the population appear in Appendix 1.

Individualized clinical data forms were designed so that all data collected were easily reduced for computer input at the time of clinic visits. Computer programs for data storage, retrieval, and analysis were developed by Frances Heide, R.N., M.S. The software package was dBaseIII on an IBM PC/XT. The software program consisted of 10 subprograms allowing the entire program to be run simultaneously with each independent subprogram using any number of selected variables. Final data analysis was done on a mainframe computer using an SAS data-analysis package.

This book is divided into two parts. Part I, Chapters 1–13, covers areas of clinical research interest, with much of the data coming from the population and methods just described. In addition, a number of the chapters contain data obtained from the individual contributor's funded grant programs. Part II, Chapters 14–19, covers selected issues and types in Down syndrome. These chapters are primarily literature reviews augmented by clinical data obtained from the described population as well as individual contributor's grant-funded research.

Don C. Van Dyke

Part I: Assessment, Characteristics, and Clinical Management in Down Syndrome

1
Common Medical Problems

DON C. VAN DYKE, DAVID J. LANG, JOHN D. MILLER,
FRANCES HEIDE, SUSAN VAN DUYNE, AND HYEJUNG CHANG

Introduction

The medical problems associated with Down syndrome have a significant impact on the delivery of all other services, whether social, educational, or developmental. The problems can be acute but are most commonly chronic, demonstrating wide variability and affecting multiple organ systems.

The medical problems of the individual with this syndrome have been studied extensively. However, it has only been in the last 20 years that aggressive medical and surgical management has become commonplace. As this trend continues, the present perspectives on the treatment of Down syndrome will change, affecting the frequency and progression of the syndrome-related disorders. Recently, with the demonstration of an Alzheimer's gene being linked to chromosome 21, molecular technology has been brought to focus on the individual with Down syndrome.

Methods and Patient Population

The demographics of the patient population in this study are outlined in the Introduction and Appendix 1. All data were reduced for computer input at the time of contact with the patient. Additional data were obtained by individual chart review of all 190 medical records. The compilation of some of this data appears in Table 1.

Review of the evaluations by the interdisciplinary team provided confirmation of the frequency of the medical and developmental problems already documented in the literature. However, a number of previously unrecognized problems were also identified and a broader perspective obtained on certain known problems. These are discussed herein.

Cardiac Abnormalities

The prevalence of cardiac disease in the Down syndrome population in the literature (40%) and in this study (33%) was similar (Greenwood & Nadas;

TABLE 1.1. Common medical problems in persons with Down syndrome (1–20 years of age).

Medical problems (history and exam)		N	Number	Percent
History of seizures		187	9	5
History of constipation		183	55	30
History of heart murmur		187	75	40
History of heart surgery		185	17	9
History of dry skin		188	74	39
Double urethral orifice	(male)	91	11	12
History of asthma		185	7	4
History of allergies		175	37	21
History of UTI/kidney infection		187	7	4
History of hair loss		178	9	5
Strabismus		150	55	37
	exotropia	(5)		
	esotropia	(50)		
Nystagmus		150	15	10
Optic nerve hypoplasia		150	16	11
Osteomyelitis		190	1	1/2
Folliculitis		190	6	3
Fungal infections		190	10	5
Pneumonia		189	57	30
Presence of significant ear wax/ear wax impaction		190	99	52
History of ear infections		189	117	62
S/P myringotomy and tubes		190	52	27
Serous otitis media		190	81	43
Sinusitis/rhinitis		190	26	14
stenotic ear canal				
Aural atresia		190	5	3

1976; Park et al., 1977; Rowe, 1962; Rowe & Uchida, 1961; Smith, 1982).

Many individuals in the study had multiple congenital cardiac defects, such as ventricular septal defect (VSD), atrial septal defect (ASD), and patent ductus arteriosus (PDA). The most common defects were VSD (20), ASD (6), and endocardial cushion/atrioventricular canal (21). There was also an increased incidence of mitral valve disorders, and of endocardial cushion defects that included mitral valve prolapse, mitral insufficiency, deformed mitral valve, and absent mitral valve. Another common defect was PDA (8). Less frequent cardiac anomalies included aortic stenosis, tetralogy of Fallot, anomalous pulmonary venous return, and pulmonary stenosis. In the younger population, cardiac catheterization had been performed in 14%; heart surgery in 9% (Table 1). The cardiac findings and management are discussed in detail in Chapter 4.

Immune Function

Pneumonia, primarily by history, had occurred at one time in 30% of this DS population. Ear infections by history were recorded in over 62%. There was an incidence of dermal folliculitis of 3–4%. Between 5 and 6% of the population had experienced fungal infections of the skin or nails. Kidney/urinary tract infections were uncommon (4%). Immunologic investigations were not performed, but the literature reports poor lymphocyte proliferation, an undefined T-cell defect, an alteration of interferon receptor function, and abnormal cell-surface receptors (Burgio et al., 1983; Levin et al., 1975). Thus, the Down syndrome population can be considered an immune compromised population.

Endocrine Dysfunction

There is a growing body of literature that suggests a higher prevalence of thyroid dysfunction in individuals with Down syndrome in comparison to a control population for age and sex. However, the clinical detection of thyroid disease, particularly hypothyroidism, is difficult because many of the clinical findings of Down syndrome are also those of hypothyroidism. In adults with this syndrome, the prevalence of hypothyroidism has been variable, ranging from 13 to 54% (Cutler, et al., 1986; Hollingsworth, et al., 1974; Murdoch et al., 1977; Quinn, 1980; Sare, et al., 1978).

In addition, adults and children with Down syndrome have an increased incidence of autoimmune disease affecting the thyroid gland and other exocrine glands (Fekete et al., 1982; Fort et al., 1984; Harris & Koutsoulieris, 1967). The incidence increases with age, requiring ongoing clinical evaluation, baseline laboratory studies, and follow-up of thyroid status.

A study of the incidence of persistent primary congenital hypothyroidism infants with Down syndrome demonstrates an incidence of 28 times that in the general population (Fort et al., 1984). The cause of thyroid aberrations in these infants, unlike that in adults, remains unclear (Fort et al., 1984). It is felt that infants with this syndrome are at high risk for congenital hypothyroidism and should have not only initial screening, but also careful and frequent follow-up.

The results of thyroid antibodies testing appear in Table 1.2. Three (2%) of 140 individuals had positive thyroglobulin antibodies. Seven (5%) had positive microsomal antibodies. In 132 individuals in whom thyroid tests for triodothyronine (T3), thyroxine (T4), and thyroid-stimulating hormone (TSH) were performed, 11 (8%) showed some abnormal thyroid value (Table 1.2). One individual had Hashimoto's thyroiditis. Two individuals showed significant elevations of TSH. Two individuals showed primary hypothyroidism with elevated TSH and low T3 and T4. There were six individuals showing varying abnormalities of thyroxine, T3, T4 and TSH requiring further evaluation including measurement of thyrotropine-releasing hormone (TRH).

Evaluation of 132 individuals with Down syndrome showed that 11 (8%) had some abnormality of thyroid function. This is considerably lower than the results of 15 to 25% reported by Pueschel and Pezzullo (1985). However, this

TABLE 1.2. Thyroid function in persons with Down syndrome.

Thyroid antibodies	
Thyroglobulin antibodies less than 1:10	137
Positive at 1:80	1
Positive at 1:60	2
	Total 140 (3)2%
Microsomal antibodies less than 1:100	132
Positive at 1:400	3
Positive at 1:1640	2
Positive at 1:6400	2
	Total 139 (7)5%

Measurement of T3, T4, TSH
Total number tested = 132

Number	*Thyroid Abnormality*
1	Hashimoto thyroiditis
2	Isolated elevation of TSH
2	Primary hypothyroidism with elevated TSH, low T3, T4
6	Abnormal T3, T4, TSH, or combination needing further evaluation
Total 11 (8%)	

is primarily a younger Down syndrome population (see Appendix 1). With increasing age there is an increasing number of thyroid abnormalities (Pueschel & Pezzullo, 1985). Among our subjects, a few individuals had normal thyroid function but elevations of thyroglobulin and microsomal antibodies. These individuals are at significant risk for future thyroid dysfunction, particularly the development of a type of thyroiditis related to Hashimoto's thyroiditis (Pueschel & Pezzullo, 1985).

Eye Conditions

There are a number of ophthalmologic, ocular, orbital, and periorbital abnormalities in individuals with Down syndrome, including variation in orbital size, abnormal palpebral fissures, and the well-known presence of epicanthal folds (Pueschel, et al., 1987; Smith & Berg, 1976; Woillez & Dansant, 1960). Parents frequently (54%) report concerns regarding eye problems/visual difficulties in this population. Lens opacities were a frequent finding in the present study, not to be confused with the 2 to 3% occurrence of cataracts (Eissler & Longenecker, 1962). Brushfield spots (30%) and blepharitis were also commonly found.

The frequent occurrence of stabismus and nystagmus in Down syndrome is well documented. These disorders may be of neuromuscular origin or due to the presence of a significant refractive error (Hiles, et al., 1974). Nystagmus was seen in 10% of this population and was most common among those children three years of age and younger. Ophthalmologic examination in these patients with Down syndrome revealed optic nerve hypoplasia and significant refractive errors. In fact, the most common and significant cause for visual loss associated with Down syndrome was refractive error (ocular conditions are detailed in Chapter 3).

Genito-urinary Tract

A significant prevalence of minor urogenital abnormalities exist in individuals with Down syndrome. The most common of these reported in the literature are microphallus and undescended testis (Smith, 1982; Smith & Berg, 1976). In a recent study, 11 of 91 males (12%) were noted to have an apparent double urethral orifice, actually a form of anterior hypospadias, an approximately 40-fold increase over reported incidence of hypospadias in the non-Down syndrome population of live born males (Lang et al., 1987). Further study revealed that the anterior orifice opened into a blind pouch while the ventral orifice was the urethral meatus leading into the bladder. Diagnostic studies did not demonstrate any anatomical abnormalities of the urethra, bladder, ureters, or kidneys. Chordee was absent in all cases (Lang et al., 1987).

With several exceptions, none of the adolescent females in this population had ever had a gynecological evaluation. Though females with Down syndrome are capable of reproduction and have given birth to both normal and trisomic infants (de La Cruz & Gerald, 1981), counseling and birth-control information had not usually been provided to a female with Down syndrome or her parents. On questioning, some parents admitted to a high level of concern regarding the potential of pregnancy; others were totally unconcerned because they believed that females with Down syndrome could not become pregnant.

Gastrointestinal Problems

The congenital abnormalities of aganglionic megacolon, duodenal obstruction due either to annular pancreas or duodenal atresia, esophageal atresia, and imperforate anus were all noted in this population of individuals (Knox & Bensel, 1972; Smith, 1982). The condition requiring the most clinical attention, however, was that of chronic constipation (30%). Due to the increased incidence of aganglionic megacolon, a few of the more severe constipation problems needed detailed diagnostic studies to rule out the possibility of an aganglionic colonic segment (Kilcoyne & Taybi, 1970; Knox & Bensel, 1972).

Feeding/Nutrition

Feeding and nutrition were common parental concerns. By report, 49% reported feeding problems with their children during the newborn period. In later life, 29% of parents had concerns about either obesity or the lack of satisfactory weight gain, with 31% reporting feeding problems. Review of newborn feeding records showed that 57% of mothers breast-fed for some significant period of time; however, bottle feeding occurred either exclusively or for some period of time in 81%.

Questions about the need for vitamin supplementation were frequently asked by parents of children with Down syndrome. Seventy-five percent of the children were on some form of multivitamin supplement. Of this group, 19% were reported to be on some type of "megavitamin therapy" program. Parents of children with Down syndrome showed a high level of interest in the use of "vitamin therapy programs," despite concerns regarding efficacy and the possibility of detrimental effects, i.e., vitamin A toxicity (Bennett et al., 1983; Smith et al., 1984).

Ear, Nose, Throat, and Hearing Disorders

Otologic problems were frequent, recurrent, and chronic in this patient population. Sixty-two percent had a history of otitis media, with 43% manifesting at one time (by history) serous otitis media (Table 1). There were a number of patients with no history of otitis media who had abnormal audiograms, with hearing loss and flat tympanograms. Hearing loss of 16dB or more in at least one ear was documented in more than 46% of this patient population. The majority of hearing loss was conductive, but a significant number of patients manifested a sensorineural hearing loss and a mixed conductive/sensorineural loss. The presence of significant impacted ear wax was a problem in at least 52% of these patients, with many needing aggressive intervention for ear wax removal (Table 1). The ENT examination showed abnormal tympanic membranes in 23%, with 7% having chronic perforated tympanic membranes. Twenty-seven percent had prior history of at least one myringotomy with the placement of tubes. Sinusitis and rhinitis were chronic problems in 14% of these patients. Clinically, the sinusitis/rhinitis responded to a 10-day course of antibiotics.

Audiograms were done on a subgroup of 60 individuals with Down syndrome. Approximately 46% of these individuals had a 16dB or greater hearing loss. The majority of hearing loss was in the mild-to-moderate range. Tympanograms showed that 43% in the right ear and 48% in the left ear had flat tympanograms (type IV curve), suggestive of middle-ear disease and/or serous fluid. Of interest was the fact that 25% of these individuals had no previous history of having had a tympanogram, nor any history of previous ear infections.

Sensory-neural, conductive, and mixed hearing losses were present in a significant number of Down syndrome individuals. Mild to moderate conductive hearing losses with type IV tympanogram curves were the most frequent findings. Of note was the fact that 25% of these individuals had no previous history of ear infections or of prior audiological evaluation. Audiologic evaluations, including tympanograms and follow-up, should be routine in these individuals, even in the absence of a history of ear problems. For a more detailed examination of hearing disorders associated with Down syndrome, see Chapter 2.

Seizures

Seizures were documented in nine individuals (5%) in this population (Table 1). The most common type of seizure experienced was infantile spasm. This observation has been previously noted in the literature (Smith & Berg, 1976).

Skin

Severe dry skin was documented in 39% of this patient population (Table 1). This problem usually responded to the use of moisturizing products such as eucerin, but a few patients needed more aggressive dermatologic intervention. Skin infections were noted in only 3 to 6%.

Musculoskeletal Problems

C1/C2 subluxation was demonstrated radiographically in 9% (i.e., 3 of 34 children, 5 to 20 years of age; see Chapter 6). This is approximately the same frequency range (10–20%) reported in the literature (Pueschel & Rynders, 1982). Because of potentially severe complications, special efforts were made to educate the parents to the precautions and management required with children with this radiographic finding. As patients grew older, radiographic examination showed an increase in degenerative disease of the cervical spine, a common finding in the adult patient with Down syndrome (Fidone, 1986).

Cancer and Leukemia

It is well known that leukemia exists more often in children with Down syndrome (Miller, 1970). It has also been suggested that these children respond poorly to chemotherapy. In general, leukemia occurs 10 to 20 times more often among children with Down syndrome than with individuals in the general population (Robinson et al., 1984). Approximately 70% of the leukemias seen are acute lymphocytic leukemia (ALL) and 30% are acute myelogenous leukemia (AML); (Miller, 1970; see Chapter 16, this volume). The peak mortality for leukemia is at one year of age; the death rate is said to be 18 times that experienced among individuals with Down syndrome (Miller, 1970).

Blood Pressure

Graphs for blood pressure were developed for both males and females for systolic and diastolic pressures (see Table 1.3). Heart rate and respiratory rate were determined for age (males and females; see Table 1.4).

TABLE 1.3. Blood pressure in Down syndrome.

Age (Months)	SYS-BP N	SYS-BP MEAN	SYS-BP STD	DIAS-BP N	DIAS-BP MEAN	DIAS-BP STD
Males						
1–23	2	70.00	14.14	2	45.00	7.07
24–29	1	95.00	—	1	50.00	—
30–35	5	89.00	2.65	5	46.00	5.48
36–41	1	90.00	—	1	40.00	—
42–47	2	90.00	14.14	2	43.00	9.90
48 +	27	94.52	10.42	26	56.08	9.83
Females						
1–23	6	78.67	14.73	6	51.00	20.70
24–29	2	86.00	5.66	2	45.00	7.07
30–35	1	84.00	—	1	36.00	—
36–41	4	84.00	11.20	4	46.50	10.75
42–47	1	82.00	—	1	48.00	—
48 +	26	90.31	14.55	26	53.81	11.10

TABLE 1.4. Pulse and respiratory rate in Down syndrome.

Age (Months)	Pulse N	Pulse MEAN	Pulse STD	Resp. Rate N	Resp. Rate MEAN	Resp. Rate STD
Males						
3–5	5	138.40	16.58	5	30.60	2.97
6–8	5	133.60	6.07	5	29.40	4.56
9–11	7	119.43	6.80	7	26.86	1.86
12–17	4	131.50	13.30	4	28.50	1.00
18–23	8	121.75	21.42	7	28.29	5.59
24–29	3	118.67	34.95	3	31.33	8.08
30–35	7	118.57	7.89	6	31.00	7.13
36–41	2	114.00	8.49	1	24.00	—
42–47	5	105.60	32.32	5	25.60	3.58
48 +	38	94.47	18.08	38	22.47	3.85
Females						
3–5	7	144.57	17.65	6	33.00	8.37
6–8	5	130.40	11.17	5	35.80	2.86
9–11	4	122.00	4.00	4	29.50	4.20
12–17	9	126.22	19.50	10	32.60	5.97
18–23	8	123.75	19.72	8	27.50	3.82
24–29	5	123.20	7.16	5	30.80	5.59
30–35	5	121.60	12.84	3	25.33	2.31
36–41	6	125.67	10.31	6	27.00	4.69
42–47	3	107.67	11.15	3	24.67	3.06
48 +	35	93.91	17.55	35	21.34	2.81

TABLE 1.5. Hematology values in Down syndrome (males and females).

	WBC			RBC			HB			HCT			PLAT		
Age (Months)	N	MEAN	STD	N	MEAN	STD	N	MEAN	STD	N	MEAN	STD	N	MEAN	STD
2	3	10.03	0.40	3	4.56	0.46	3	14.90	1.68	3	45.13	5.88	3	327.67	64.53
3	2	8.25	1.34	2	4.37	1.07	2	13.55	3.61	2	41.25	12.09	1	370.00	—
4	4	6.75	1.71	4	3.93	0.55	4	11.87	2.07	4	36.85	5.63	4	602.00	167.80
5	6	8.75	5.20	6	4.31	0.56	6	12.40	1.06	6	36.97	3.47	6	487.33	77.75
6–23	35	7.59	2.91	35	4.38	0.46	35	13.15	1.43	35	39.89	4.67	33	403.67	120.47
24–47	35	6.64	1.88	35	4.23	0.37	35	12.62	0.87	35	38.27	2.95	34	378.76	82.31
48+	69	6.52	2.11	69	4.45	0.43	69	13.88	1.41	69	42.18	4.50	63	353.14	114.09

Hematology

Hematology values were calculated using the complete blood count results of 74 males and 80 females with Down syndrome for white blood cells, red blood cell count, hemaglobin, hematocrit, and platelets. These values appear in Table 1.5.

Allergy

Parents gave a positive response to allergies to food/medication or a positive allergy history like allergic rhinitis in 21% (37). Hair loss probably on an autoimmune basis was seen in 5% (9). A history of asthma was reported in only 4% (7).

Summary

The trend toward deinstitutionalization of persons with Down syndrome has resulted in the greater involvement of parents in their care, and the increasing contact of these children with primary care practitioners. As a result there is a greater need for primary care practitioners to understand and recognize the common medical problems and needs of the child and young adult who has this syndrome. As time goes on, the use of computerized data retrieval will allow for the collection of relevant statistics, the establishment of clinical correlations, and the study of the multiple medical problems that often accompany Down syndrome, including those associated with growth and nutrition, hearing and speech disorders, foot and gait abnormalities, endocrinopathies, immune deficiency, cardiac and gastrointestinal disturbances, infections, diseases, ophthalmological problems, and dental and craniofacial abnormalities (some of these are listed in Table 1.1).

As expert primary medical care for these individuals becomes increasingly available, their mean life expectancy will continue to increase, with more and more children surviving to adulthood. The concerns of pediatricians will become the problems of internists and family practice physicians. It should be a natural development that interdisciplinary programs will be extended to serve the needs of adults with Down syndrome and to provide support and education for the relevant health care personnel who will provide primary medical care for these individuals.

It should also be noted that economic factors play a crucial role in determining the success and ultimately even the feasibility of interdisciplinary programs. Third-party coverage is not always widely available for primary preventive health care for children with developmental disabilities. The provision or lack of coverage by third-party payers for preventive health care for these high-risk individuals may ultimately determine whether efforts to limit the progression of their disabilities, to maximize their potential as citizens, will be possible.

References

Bennett, F.C., McClelland, S., Kriesgsmann, E.A., Andrus, L.B., & Sells, C.J. (1983). Vitamin and mineral supplementation in Down's syndrome. *Pediatrics, 72*(5), 707–713.

Burgio, G.R., Ugazio, A., Nespoli, L., & Maccario, R. (1983). Down syndrome: A model of immunodeficiency. *Birth Defects* (Original article series), *19*(3), 325–327

Cutler, A.T., Benezra-Obeiter, R., & Brink, S.J. (1986). Thyroid function in young children. *American Journal of Diseases of Children, 140*, 479–483.

de la Cruz, F.F., & Gerald, P.S. (Eds.). (1981). *Trisomy 21 (Down syndrome) Research Perspective.* Baltimore: University Park Press.

Eissler, R., & Longenecker, L.P. (1962). The common eye findings in mongolism. *American Journal of Ophthalmology, 54*, 398–406.

Fekete, G., Kulcsar, G., Dann, P., Nasz, I., Schuler, D., & Dobos, M. (1982). Immunological and virological investigations in Down's syndrome. *European Journal of Pediatrics, 138*, 59–62.

Fidone, G.S. (1986). Degenerative cervical arthritis in Down syndrome. *New England Journal of Medicine, 312* (5), 320.

Fort, P., Lifschitz, F., Bellisario, R., Davis, J., Lanes, R., Pugliese, M., Richman, R., Post, E.M., & David, R. (1984). Abnormalities of thyroid function in infants with Down syndrome. *Journal of Pediatrics, 104* (4), 545–549.

Greenwood, R.D., & Nadas, A.S. (1976). The clinical course of cardiac disease in Down's syndrome. *Pediatrics, 58*(6), 893–897.

Harris, F., & Koutsoulieris, E. (1967). Hypothyroidism due to autoimmune thyroiditis in a young child with Down syndrome. *Archives of Disease of Childhood, 42*, 449–452.

Hiles, D.A., Hoyme, S.H., & McFarlane, F. (1974). Down's syndrome and strabismus. *American Orthoptic Journal, 24*, 63–68.

Hollingsworth, D.E., McKean, H.E., & Roekel, I. (1974). Goiter, immunological observations and thyroid function tests in Down syndrome. *American Journal of Diseases of Children, 127*, 524–527.

Kilcoyne, R.F., & Taybi, H. (1970). Conditions associated with congenital megacolon. *American Journal of Roentgen Radium Thermal Nuclear Medicine, 108*, 615–620.

Knox, G.E., & Bensel, R.W. (1972). Gastrointestinal malformations in Down syndrome. *Minnesota Medicine, 55*, 542–545.

Lang, D.J., Van Dyke, D.C., Heide, F., & Lowe, P.L. (1987). Hypospadia and urethral abnormalities in Down syndrome. *Clinical Pediatrics, 26* (1), 40–42.

Levin, S., Nir, E., & Mogilner, B.M. (1975). T-system immune deficiency in Down's syndrome. *Pediatrics, 56*, 123–126.

Miller, R.W. (1970). Neoplasia and Down's syndrome. *Annual New York Academy of Science, 171*, 637–644.

Murdoch, J.C., et al. (1977). Thyroid function in adults with Down syndrome. *Journal of Clinical Endocrinology, 44*, 453–458.

Park, S.C., Mathews, R.A., Zuberbuhler, J.R., Rowe, R.D., Neches, W.H., & Lenox, C.C. (1977). Down syndrome with congenital heart disease. *American Journal of Diseases of Children, 131*, 29–33.

Pueschel, S.M., & Pezzullo, J.C. (1985). Thyroid dysfunction in Down syndrome. *American Journal of Diseases of Children, 139*, 636–639.

Pueschel, S.M., & Rynders, T.E. (1982). *Down syndrome: Advances in biomedicine and the behavioral sciences* (pp. 243–246). Mass: Cambridge, Ware Press.

Pueschel, S.M., Tingey, C., Rynders, J.E., Crocker, A.C., & Crutcher, D.M. (1987). *New perspectives on Down syndrome*. Baltimore: Paul H. Brookes.

Quinn, M.W. (1980). Down syndrome and hypothyroidism. *Journal of Medical Science, 1*, 19–22.

Resner, F., & Lee, S.L. (1972). Down's syndrome and acute leukemia: Myeloblastic or lymphocytic? Report of forty-three cases and review of the literature. *American Journal of Medicine, 53* (2), 203–218.

Robinson, L.L., et al. (1984). Down syndrome and acute leukemia in children: A ten-year retrospective survey from children's cancer study group. *Journal of Pediatrics, 105*, 235–242.

Rowe, D. (1962). Cardiac malformation in mongolism. *American Heart Journal, 64*, 567–569.

Rowe, R.D., & Uchida, I.A. (1961). Cardiac malformation in mongolism: A prospective study of 184 mongoloid children. *American Journal of Medicine, 31*, 726–735.

Sare, Z., Recvalcaba, R.H.A., & Kelley, V.C. (1978). Prevalence of thyroid disorders in Down syndrome. *Clinical Genetics, 14*, 154–158.

Smith, D.W. (1982). *Recognizable patterns of human malformations*. Philadelphia: W.B. Saunders.

Smith, G.F., Spiker, D., Peterson, C.P., Cicchetti, D. & Justine, P. (1984). Use of megadoses of vitamins with minerals in Down syndrome. *Journal of Pediatrics, 105* (2), 228–234.

Smith, G.R., & Berg, J.M. (1976). *Down's anomaly*, 2d ed. New York: Churchill-Livingstone.

Woillez, M., & Dansant, C. (1960). *Les manifestations occulaires dans le mongolisme. Archive of Ophthalmology* (Paris), *20*, 810–828.

2
Ear, Nose, and Throat Problems and Hearing Abnormalities

DON C. VAN DYKE, MAURICE E. POPEJOY, AND
WILLIAM G. HEMENWAY

Introduction

Ear, nose, oral, pharyngeal, and hearing problems are frequent areas of concern in children with Down syndrome. From a management standpoint, recurrent ear infections with associated hearing loss, chronic sinusitis with rhinorrhea, and ear wax impaction are frequent primary care concerns and often require long-term medical intervention and follow-up. Frequently reported anomalies of the palate, midface, and external auditory canals often involve both medical and surgical management issues.

Children with Down syndrome are known to have a high prevalence of hearing loss (Balkany, Downs, et al., 1979). In one series of 107 individuals with this syndrome, significant hearing loss was found in about two-thirds of the patients (Balkany, et al., 1979). The incidence of hearing loss recorded varies from study to study, ranging from 42 to 77%, but all studies show a significant increase of hearing impairment over that of the general population (Brooks, et al., 1972; Fulton & Lloyd, 1968; Glovsky, 1966).

Common Ear, Nose, and Throat (ENT) Problems

Abnormal Palate

High-arch palate has been listed as a typical finding in Down syndrome by some authors (Levinson, et al., 1955). However, recent reviewers feel that the term "high-arch palate" is more commonly a manifestation of a subjective, rather than an objective, clinical observation. Recent measurements of palates in persons with Down syndrome (Redman, et al., 1965) have suggested that high-arched and narrow palates are not characteristic of this syndrome. While the palates of adults with Down syndrome appear to be appreciably smaller in all dimensions than those of normal adults, they are not unusually high-arched.

It has been documented that clefts of the palate occur with a frequency greater in individuals with Down syndrome than in the general population, with a reported range of 0.2 to 5%. Studies by Schendel and Gorlin (1974) estimated that the frequency of cleft palate in association with Down syndrome was 4.6%, while that of submucous cleft was 0.78%.

Noisy Breathing

Items of frequent report by parents of children with Down syndrome are noisy breathing, abnormal respiratory patterns, and mouth breathing. It has been demonstrated that the incidence of hypernasality in this syndrome is higher than that of the general population. In a study by Kavanagh, Kahane, and Kordan (1986) it was demonstrated in 6 of 21 patients who presented with mouth breathing, tongue protrusion, and snorting, sleep apnea was present. Thus, in the child with the significant facial features of Down syndrome, an abnormal sleep pattern, nasal breathing, and obesity, sleep apnea must also be a consideration.

Sinusitis

Purulent rhinorrhea, sometimes with sinusitis, is a frequent presentation of Down syndrome. In one study, 40% of Down syndrome patients had prevalent rhinorrhea on examination (Strome, 1981). Adenoidectomy appeared to have no effect; allergies did not appear to be playing a role. Nasal cultures taken from these patients did not demonstrate a predominant organism. Treatment with low-dosage ampicillin, 250 mg twice a day in children over two years of age and 125 mg twice a day in children under two years of age, resulted in resolution of the rhinorrhea in 9 of 10 cases.

External Ear and External Auditory Canal

Children with Down syndrome show deficient growth in craniofacial structures, including maldevelopment of the external ear. A study by Aase, Wilson, and Smith (1973) showed that in children with Down syndrome from birth to one year of age the size of ear length or longitudinal dimension of the pinna was more than two standard deviations below the norm. In older children and adults, the length was more variable but consistently at least one standard deviation or more below the norm.

The external auditory canals of individuals with Down syndrome have been noted to be small. In a study by Strome, 70 to 80% had small canals, while 39% had some degree of canal stenosis. In addition, other growth abnormalities have been noted, including cochleosaccular dysplasia (Walby & Schuknecht, 1984) and ossicular abnormalities (Balkany, Mischke, et al., 1979). An analysis of the temporal bones in children with Down syndrome has revealed multiple middle ear abnormalities, including fixation of the stapes, structural deformation of the stapes, and dehiscence of the facial canal

(Balkany, Mischke, et al., 1979). It is felt that congenital external auditory canal atresia or stenosis is not the same type of ear canal stenosis seen in children with Down syndrome who have smaller ear canals but not atretic plates or absent typanic membranes (Grundfast & Camilon, 1986).

Cerumen

Down syndrome individuals have increased incidence of excessive accumulation of cerumen. In a study by Dahle and McCollister (1986), impaction of cerumen and other debris was found to be a frequent medical problem. Those individuals with ear wax impaction had hearing losses averaging 24 dB.

Otitis Media

Otitis media is highly prevalent among children with Down syndrome. In a study by Schwartz and Schwartz (1978) of institutionalized Down syndrome patients, it was found that 59% had at least a unilateral middle ear effusion. The incidence was higher, reaching 80% in children with stenotic external auditory canals. In a study by Samuelson and Nguyen (1980) of 138 patients with Down syndrome, 39% had ear disease, with 63% having middle ear effusion. Of that 63%, 40% were treated medically, and 60% by myringotomies and tubes. In a survey of 107 children with Down syndrome, bilateral hearing loss was noted in 64%, with 78% having hearing loss in one or both ears (Balkany, Downs et al., 1979). It is felt by some that children with Down syndrome are significantly affected by sensory deprivation, and that these children in particular need preventive measures if they are to reach their full cognitive potential (Balkany, Downs et al., 1979).

For some individuals having Down syndrome, myringotomies and tubes provide effective relief in cases of serous otitis media. Despite this treatment, however, 14% were estimated to have recurrences (Downs et al., 1981). Some authors feel that any language delay in children with this syndrome should be promptly treated with a home language-stimulation program, and where hearing loss is more extensive, amplification using a hearing aid (Downs et al., 1981).

Hearing Abnormalities

There is some discussion about what constitutes a significant hearing loss; however, most researchers accept a hearing loss in which the threshold of hearing is, on the average, greater than 15 dB as significant (Downs, 1977: Holm & Kunze, 1969; Kessner et al., 1974). In a study by Balkany, Downs, et al. (1979), 78% of persons examined had a significant hearing loss, and 83% of these losses were conductive. Of greater importance was the fact that 64% of these subjects had binaural hearing loss (Balkany, Downs, et al. 1979). Thus, hearing loss must be viewed as an important health problem in the child with Down syndrome. In an institutionalized population of children and young adults with this syndrome, a large number showed hearing impairments with a conductive loss (Fulton et al., 1964). Recent studies by Maurizi et al. (1985) reinforce the fact that middle ear pathology and associated hearing loss in Down syndrome is more frequent than would be expected in the general population. In children where impedance testing and sound field evaluation cannot be reliably tested, brainstem audiometry should be a major consideration (Maurizi et al., 1985). While impedance tests are most accurate in detection of middle ear pathology, auditory evoked response (ABR) is the most reliable tool in threshold definition, allowing a differential diagnosis between sensorineural and moderate conductive hearing loss (Paludetti et al., 1979).

Audiological evaluation in adults with Down syndrome presents a picture similar to that of children. In a study of 51 subjects, 51 to 74% had some degree of hearing impairment (Keiser, et al., 1981). Thus, the adult continues to show an ongoing picture of frequent ear problems and chronic hearing loss.

While Down syndrome has been associated with conductive hearing loss and otitis media, additional studies have shown other abnormalities leading to significant hearing loss. A study by Balkany, Mischky et al. (1979) showed a frequency in Down syndrome of middle ear abnormalities including fixation and superstructure deformity of the stapes, and dehiscence of the facial canal. Other studies have shown inner ear abnormalities such as cochleosaccular dysplasia with a short cochlea and small lateral semicircular canal in patients with profound deafness (Walby & Schuknecht, 1984).

In summary, adults and children with Down syndrome have an increased prevalence of hearing loss with hearing thresholds of greater than 15 dB. There is an increase in conductive hearing loss due to recurrent otitis media, and serous otitis on a chronic basis. In addition, a small but significant number have, in conjunction with their conductive hearing loss, a sensory-neural hearing loss, due in some cases, to inner ear anomalies. Thus, the audiological evaluation of the individual with Down syndrome must be aggressive and thorough, and should, when indicated, include ABR.

The management of hearing loss with the person who has this syndrome should be equally aggressive (Downs et al., 1981). Medical and surgical treatment (myringotomies and tubes) should be used appropriately. After three months duration of serous otitis media, a language evaluation should be performed (Downs et al., 1981). Any language delay should be managed appropriately. Children with Down syndrome are "otitis prone," have an increased prevalence of hearing loss, and have cognitive and auditory perceptual problems. Thus, they are at significant risk for delay in their language development.

ENT Population

We reviewed the case histories, including medical and ENT examinations of 190 individuals with Down syndrome. The demographics of this population are presented in Appendix 1. Parents of each individual were asked to complete a questionnaire. Specific areas in which questions were asked were: history of otitis media, history of myringotomies and tubes, history of recurrent serous otitis media, the presence on examination of abnormal tympanic membranes (i.e., perforation), the presence of earwax, and the presence of stenotic ear canals.

All 190 individuals were seen in an interdisciplinary clinic, some on multiple occasions. They were evaluated by a ENT physician and by a pediatrician with an interest in pediatric ENT. The results of the ENT findings were recorded.

Audiology Population

A subgroup of 132 individuals of the 190 seen in ENT clinics were given tympano grams. Of these 132 individuals, 60 children were evaluated under head phones to determine pure tone thresholds and speech reception thresholds.

Equipment and Methods

Equipment

The audiologic evaluations were completed in a single wall 10-foot-by-10-foot sound room, Tracoustics model RE-144. The ambient noise levels in the test room met permissible octave-band levels for background noise for audiometric testing rooms (pure tone air, bone, and sound field diagnostic testing).

A Madsen OB-822 diagnostic clinical audiometer was calibrated to ANSI S3.6 1969 standards. The audiometer was electroacoustically calibrated and rectified quarterly. Additionally, the audiometer calibration was verified biologically each day of use. A CyberSmith visual reinforcement system was used as the reinforcer for the Visual Reinforcement Audiometry (VRA). An EVE II (American-Electromedics) clinical tympanometer was used for the middle ear impedance measurements.

A well equipped pediatric ENT facility was available, with the appropriate equipment for evaluating persons whose ages ranged from newborns to adults. The examination was aided by an operating room microscope located in the outpatient clinic.

Methods

1. The ENT evaluation was conducted using standard pediatric ENT equipment, plus an operating room microscope. Physical assessment of the head and neck region were included as part of this evaluation; results appear in Table 2.1. Some children needed to be seen several times for ear wax removal. Many of the children needed multiple treatments with mineral oil

TABLE 2.1. Physical characteristics of the head and neck in Down syndrome.

Physical characteristics	Number of individuals examined	Characteristic	% of total
Head size (microcephaly)	176	105	60
Midfacial hypoplasia	180	160	89
Depressed nasal bridge	180	149	83
Hypertelorism	180	14	8
Small pinna	178	138	78
Over-folded helix	179	125	70
Low-set ears	180	9	5

or Debox®, and some needed several sessions for total cleansing of the external auditory canal and visualization of the tympanic membrane. The accumulated wax was a significant cause of hearing loss.

2. Pure tone threshold testing was accomplished under headphones or by bone conduction using play audiometry. The speech reception thresholds were obtained using live voice speech and selected spondee words taken from the guidelines for determining the threshold level, either using speech or pointing to body parts (ASHA, 1979). Speech discrimination was not assessed in these children.
3. The behavioral sound field evaluations were accomplished using visual reinforcement audiometry (VRA), and the child's responses were compared to the Auditory Behavior Index (Northern & Downs, 1984). The developmental age for the child was established using the Rapid Developmental Screening Checklist. Children who could not be conditioned to VRA were excluded from this study. The severity levels for the sound field evaluations were based on the apparent developmental age and the child's minimal response level.

Results

Review of ENT history questionnaires given to 190 parents of individuals having Down syndrome showed that 32% had a history of hearing impairments, with 62% giving a positive history of recurrent ear infections (Table 2.2). On ENT examination, and/or by history, it was noted that at least 31% had experienced at least one episode of otitis media (Table 2.3). Documented by examination and/or tympanograms, more than 43% have, or had previously, serous otitis media. At least 27% of this population have had myringotomies and tubes at least once (Table 2.3).

Evaluation of the tympanic membranes of these individuals frequently showed evidence of otitis media, serous otitis media, and/or small ear canals. In 3% of this population the external ear canals so narrow that the tympanic membranes could not be visualized. Abnormal tympanic membranes, other

TABLE 2.2. Ear, nose, throat history.

Problem area	N	Individuals with positive history	% of total
Hearing impairment	174	56	32
Recurrent ear infection	189	117	62
Pneumonia	189	57	30
Allergies	175	37	21
Difficulties in talking	168	93	55

N = Number of complete questionnaire responses by parents of 190 individuals with Down syndrome.

TABLE 2.3. Ear, nose, throat abnormalities in Down syndrome. Total number = 190 individuals.

Age in years	0–1	1–3	3–5	5–12	12–21	Total	%
Ears							
Otitis media	9	25	6	12	7	59	31
S/P myringotomy & tubes (history)	4	12	8	18	10	52	27
Serous otitis media (history)	18	26	13	20	4	81	43
Abnormal membrane (by exam)	16	21	5	5	1	48	25
Ear wax (by exam)	22	28	18	19	12	99	52
Stenotic ear canals (by exam)	—	—	2	2	1	5	3
Oral Cavity							
Constricted palate	13	21	6	7	3	50	26
Submucous cleft	—	—	—	1	—	1	< 1
Sleep apnea (evaluation)	1	—	—	1	1	3	2
Sinuses							
Sinusitis/rhinorrhea	2	7	4	9	4	26	14

than those with otitis media and/or serous otitis media, were noted in 25%. The most common tympanic membrane findings were tympanosclerosis or perforation (Table 2.2).

Upper respiratory infections and pneumonias appeared to be frequent in this population, occurring in at least 30% of individuals (Table 2.2). Sinusitis with rhinorrhea was also a common finding (14%); those so diagnosed were treated medically, in most cases with amoxicillin, usually with resolution of the rhinorrhea (Table 2.3).

There were no occurrences of cleft lip or bifid uvula, but one patient was noted to have a submucous cleft. Noisy breathing or mouth breathing were noted frequently on examination, but only three individuals (2%) were documented on evaluation as having sleep apnea (Table 2.3)

Ear wax buildup was a major problem with these children. It was the most frequently noted problem on examination, with 52% showing significant ear

TABLE 2.4. Hearing in Down syndrome.

Hearing loss[a]	Right ear N(60)		Left ear N(60)		Sound field N(48)	
dB-HL	Number	(%)	Number	(%)	Number	(%)
0–15	32	(53)	31	(52)	23	(48)
16–25	13	(22)	11	(18)	13	(27)
26–40	8	(13)	10	(17)	9	(19)
41–55	1	(2)	4	(7)	3	(6)
56–70	3	(5)	2	(3)	0	(0)
71–90	0	—	0	—	0	(0)
90+	3	(5)	2	(3)	0	(0)

[a]Hearing loss (dB-HL) represents a three frequency pure tone average.

TABLE 2.5. Tympanograms.

	Right ear			Left ear		
Type of tympanogram	N tested	[a]	% of[a]	N tested	[a]	% of[a]
Normal	35	8	23	33	7	21
Reduced compliance and normal pressure	3	0	—	4	0	—
Hypermobility and normal pressure	1	0	—	0	0	—
Flat tympanogram	56	14	25	63	16	25
Normal compliance with negative pressure	18	4	22	17	3	18
Physical volume test consistent with perforation or patent tube	18	1	6	15	1	6
Total	131			132		

[a]Individuals with no previous tympanogram or history of previous ear infections.

wax that required removal. Determination of this diagnosis was aided in part by the use of the operating room microscope. In some patients wax had never been removed and was impacted and difficult to extract.

The hearing of 60 of these 131 children was evaluated using headphones. Pure tone thresholds and speech reception thresholds were obtained for both ears. Forty-eight percent of these children had significant hearing loss, with a pure tone average of 16 dB or greater. The majority were in the mild to moderate range (Table 2.4).

Forty-eight children with Down syndrome were evaluated in a sound field using a VRA technique, and the response considered is that of the best hearing ear. Fifty-two percent of these children's minimal response levels were judged to indicate significant hearing loss greater than 16 dB when compared with Baby Auditory Behavior Index (BABI) at their developmental age. Out of 190 individuals, tympanograms were obtained on 131 right ears and 132 left ears (Table 2.5). A satisfactory tympanogram of the right ear was not obtainable on one person in the study.

Discussion

Otitis media appears to be a frequent problem in Down syndrome. The most common outcomes of this diagnosis include hearing loss, speech delay, serous otitis media, tympanosclerosis, and, in a few cases, chronic ear problems with tympanic membrane perforation. Small ear canals are a frequent finding in conjunction with Down syndrome; however, only 3% were noted to have ear canals stenotic to the extent that the tympanic membrane could not be seen. The presence of small ear canals made ear wax removal a major problem. At least 52% of the children needed aggressive medical management of their ear wax buildup. It is felt that the prophylactic use of ear wax softeners should be a consideration in the treatment of all individuals with this syndrome, for the presence of ear wax can have a significant effect on hearing; one study reporting an average loss of 24 db (Dahle & McCollister, 1986). For this reason, management of ear wax problems needs to be an ongoing effort. Sinusitis also appears to be a frequent problem, appearing in 14% of this population. All cases were treated medically, using oral antibiotics, with resolution.

These data (52% with hearing loss) support the findings of earlier studies (Balkany, Downs, et al., 1979; Keiser et al., 1981) which showed hearing loss in the Down syndrome population of 40–78%. Of interest in this study is the use of a tympanogram as a screening device for all individuals with Down syndrome, regardless of history, and the fact that 25% of the individuals tested had flat tympanograms, but nonetheless had no previous history of a tympanogram or any history of ear infection. The findings of a flat tympanogram is in line with the number of individuals with hearing loss (43 to 48% versus 46%). Clearly, the absence of a history of ear infection is not a good indicator of normal hearing. A number of persons with Down syndrome are "otitis prone" with serous otitis media, but are not being diagnosed and treated. Frequent testing and follow-up are needed. The results of a hearing history questionnaire (Table 2.6) continue to support these findings; this high-risk population is not being referred for audiologic evaluation early in life.

TABLE 2.6. Hearing questionnaire administered to parents of children with Down syndrome.

History	N	Yes response	%
Prior infections	166	90	54
No prior infections[a]	166	76	46
Prior audiologic evaluation	166	92	55
No prior audiologic evaluation	166	74	45

[a]Of the 74 Down syndrome children who had no prior audiologic evaluations, 57 (70%) were younger than three years old.

Summary

Children with Down syndrome demonstrate significant ENT problems, primarily recurrent otitis media, that may require both surgical and medical management. Ear wax buildup with impaction is an ongoing outpatient management problem. Though constricted palates and submucous clefts have been reported in the past, they were not areas of major concern in this population. The sinusitis/rhinnorrhea that was diagnosed responded to appropriate medical management.

The absence of a history or physical findings of ear infections is not a good indicator of normal hearing. A number of individuals with Down syndrome who have serous otitis media are not being diagnosed and treated. Frequent audiologic testing and follow-up is needed.

References

Aase, J.M., Wilson, A.C., & Smith, D.W. (1973). Small ears in Down's syndrome: A helpful diagnostic aid. *Journal of Pediatrics, 82* (5), 845–847.

American Speech, Hearing and Language Association (ASHA). (1979). Guidelines for determining the threshold level of speech, *Journal of American Speech, Language and Hearing Association, 21* (5), 353–356.

Balkany, T.J., Downs, M.P., Jafek, B.W., & Krajicek, M.J. (1979). Hearing loss in Down's syndrome: A treatable handicap more common than generally recognized. *Clinical Pediatrics, 18* (2), 116–118.

Balkany, T.J., Mischke, R.E., Downs, M.P., & Jafek, B.W. (1979). Ossicular abnormalities in Down's syndrome. *Otolaryngology Head and Neck Surgery, 87*, 372–384.

Brooks, D.N., Wooley, A., & Kanjilal, G.C. (1972). Hearing loss and middle ear disorders in patients with Down's syndrome (Mongolism). *Journal of Mental Deficiency Research, 16*, 21.

Dahle, A.J., & McCollister, F.P. (1986). Hearing and otologic disorders in children with Down' syndrome. *American Journal of Mental Deficiency, 90*, 636–642.

Downs, M.P. (1977). The expanding imperatus of early identification. *Childhood deafness: Causation, assessment and management*, F.H. Bess (Ed.), New York: Grune & Stratton.

Downs, M.P., Jafek, B.W., & Wood, II, R.P. (1981). Comprehensive treatment of children with recurrent serous otitis media. *Otolaryngology Head and Neck Surgery, 89*, 658–665.

Fulton, R., & Lloyd, L. (1968). Hearing impairment in a population of children with Down's syndrome. *American Journal of Mental Deficiency, 73*, 298–302.

Glovsky, L. (1966). Audiological assessment of a mongoloid population. *Training School Bulletin, 33*, 37.

Grundfast, K.M., & Camilon, F. (1986). External auditory canal stenosis in palatal atresia without associated anomalies. *Annals of Otorhinolaryngology, 95*, 505–509.

Holm, V., & Kunze, L. (1969). Effect of chronic otitis media on language and speech development. *Pediatrics, 43*, 883.

Kavanagh, K.T., Kahane, K.C., & Kordan, B. (1986). Risk and benefits of adenotonsilectomy for children with Down's syndrome. *American Journal of Mental Deficiency, 91* (1), 22–29.

Keiser, H., Montague, J., Wold, D., Maune, S., & Pattison, S.M. (1981). Hearing loss of Down syndrome adults. *American Journal of Mental Deficiency, 85* (5), 467–472.

Kessner, D.M., Snow, C.K., & Singer, J. (1974). Assessment of medical care for children. *Contrasts in Health Status Vol. III.* Washington, D.C.: National Academy of Science.

Levinson, A., Friedman, A., & Stamps, F. (1955). Variability of Mongolism. *Pediatrics, 16*, 43.

Maurizi, M., Ottaviani, F., Paludetti, G., & Lungarotti, S. (1985). Audiological findings in Down's syndrome. *International Journal of Pediatric Otorhinolaryngology, 9*, 227–232.

Northern, J.L., & Downs, M.P. (1984). *Hearing in children*, 3d ed. Baltimore, Md.: Williams and Wilkins.

Paludetti, G., Maurizi, M., Altissimi, G., Frenguelli, A., Ottaviani, F., & Rosignolli, M. (1979). L'audiometria del tronco dell' encefalo in alcuni tipi di ipoacusie-perifericche. *Nuovo Arch It Otol., 7*, 519–542.

Redman, R.S., Shapiro, B.L., & Gorlin, R.J. (1965). Measurement of normal and reportedly malformed palatal vaults III, Down syndrome (trisomy 21, mongolism). *Journal of Pediatrics, 67* (2), 162–165.

Samuelson, M.E., & Nguyen, V.T. (1980). Middle ear effusion in Down's syndrome patients. *Nebraska Medical Journal, 65* (4), 83–84.

Schendel, S.A., & Gorlin, R.J. (1974). Frequency of cleft uvula and submucous cleft in patients with Down's syndrome. *Journal of Dental Research, 53* (4), 840–843.

Schwartz, D.M., & Schwartz, R.H. (1978). Acoustic impedance and otoscopic findings in children with Down's syndrome. *Archives of Otolaryngology, 104* (11), 652–656.

Strome, M. (1981). Down's syndrome: A modern otorhinolaryngological perspective. *The Laryngoscope, 91* (10), 1581–1594.

Walby, A.P., & Schuknecht, H.F. (1984). Concomitant occurrence of cochleoccular dysplasia in Down's syndrome. *Archives of Otolaryngology, 110* (7), 447–479.

3
Ophthalmological Aspects

WALTER M. FIERSON

Introduction

Unusual characteristics of the eye were among the earliest recognized features of Down syndrome; a typical periocular appearance was first described by Langdon Down in his initial report on the subject in 1986. The superficial resemblance of these ocular characteristics to those of some oriental peoples was noted by some authors, giving rise to the alternative name for the syndrome, "Mongolism." These observations of periocular morphologic change were the cornerstone of a Darwinian theory of "racial regression," proposed by Down to explain causation of the syndrome. This theory was later disproven when Lejuene, Gauthier, and Turpin (1959) reported on the specific chromosome anomaly, trisomy 21.

As with the systemic anomalies found in other tissues and organ systems in patients with Down syndrome, the ocular changes wrought by the additional genetic material are quite prevalent, including some of the most frequently noted alternations in this syndrome, and variable in incidence, severity, and profundity of functional impact. An informed diagnostic approach and early therapeutic intervention can prevent almost all visual loss; the blindness frequently reported in past times is usually avoidable with proper care and follow-up and patient educability can be significantly improved by minimizing visual loss. Pediatric ophthalmologic examination techniques can be applied readily to patients with Down syndrome, so that patients of any age can, and should, be examined. Therapy can thus be instituted in a timely fashion.

Patient Population

The information presented in this chapter derives from two sources: patients who were personally studied by the author, and additional data culled from the medical literature. The 150 patients in this study present the largest study group of patients with Down syndrome reported in the ophthalmologic medical literature. They were gathered from two sources: 101 patients were from a Down syndrome study group screened at the City of Hope National Medical Center in California, and a second group of 49 patients from the private practice of the author. These two groups were alike in that all patients were referred to the author for ophthalmologic screening. Other patients with Down syndrome referred to the author for treatment of specific ophthalmologic disorders were excluded from this study to avoid the creation of statistical bias.

Methods

All patients were examined and treated by the author. The study was prospective only in the sense that the intent to study the group was present prior to examining them, and a standardized examination was performed on all patients. Six individuals, insufficiently cooperative for performance of this examination, were excluded from the study. Each patient was examined in the following manner: Visual acuity was evaluated by binocular fixation pattern, Allen symbols, or Snellen letters; the particular method used was dependent on the patient's age and mental capacity. Pupillary testing, including tests for afferent pupillary defect, was performed with fixation at distance (Solomons et al., 1965). Occular mobility testing was performed by standard cover testing with accommodation controlled by age-appropriate distant and near fixation targets or toys. Eyelid examination was accomplished by direct inspection and slit lamp examination; Marginal blepharitis was diagnosed by either technique when characteristic scaling and inflammation of the eyelid margins were present. Anterior segment evaluation was carried out by using a standard fixed slit lamp biomicroscope or a hand-held slit lamp microscope. Retinoscopy was carried out under cyclopentolate cyclopegia with fixation controlled by distant fixation targets using a Copeland streak retinoscope. Fundus examinations were performed using indirect ophthalmoscopy after sufficient pupillary dilation was achieved with cyclopentolate. Criteria used for diagnosis of specific conditions is noted in the sections of the chapter dealing with those entities. A control group consisted of 100 consecutive non–Down patients referred for routine ophthalmologic screening during the time period of this study.

Background

Eyelid Morphology

No physical findings were felt to be more characteristic of Down syndrome than the associated eyelid anomalies; indeed, it was these anomalies that initially led Langdon Down to split off one group of persons with mental retardation from the larger population of his patients into a distinct diagnostic subgroup (Down, 1866).

A great deal of descriptive material regarding the eyelid morphology in Down syndrome patients is present in the literature. Unfortunately, this material has been subject to very scant quantification. It is certainly the feeling of most workers in the field that the eyelids of patients with this syndrome are quite characteristic, but what has not been explicitly stated is that the lid configuration of patients with this syndrome is strikingly similar. The characteristics most frequently put forth as symptomatic of Down syndrome included: obliquity of the palpebral fissure, decreased length of the palpebral fissure, epicanthal folds, telecanthus, and symmetry of curvature of the upper eyelid. Aside from morphological characteristics, it has been reported that marginal blepharitis is quite common in patients with Down syndrome (Down, 1866; Solomons et al., 1965; Eissler & Longenscher, 1962; Lowe, 1949; Lyle et al., 1972; Shapiro & France, 1985).

A slanted palpebral fissure is quite common in Down syndrome. Palpebral fissure slant may be defined as the variation from horizontal of a line drawn from the medial canthus to the lateral canthus. This may be measured by means of a modified protractor reported by Shapiro and France (1985), or by measurement of the height of the lateral canthus above the medial canthus directly in millimeters, with conversion into angular deviation by trigonometric means. Using their protractor, Shapiro and France found that 89% of a population of 53 patients with Down syndrome had a palpebral fissure slant of 6 degrees or more, while 100% of control subjects had a palpebral fissure inclination of 5 degrees or less.

Mongoloid slant was defined as that angle present when the outer canthus is higher than the inner canthus, and anti-Mongoloid slant is where the inner canthus is higher than the outer canthus. Solomons et al. (1965) found a Mongoloid slant of the eyes in 60% of 138 institutionalized individuals having Down syndrome, and in 94% of 78 noninstitutionalized individuals with Down syndrome who were under the age of 10 years Table 3.1.

A Mongoloid slant was present in 14% of control individuals. However, the slant was defined as being significant if the outer canthus was more than 2 mil-

TABLE 3.1. Structural eyelid abnormalities in Down syndrome.

Palpebral fissure obliquity
Epicanthal folds
Diminished palpebral fissure length
Symmetrical upper eyelid curvature
Possible nasolacrimal duct obstruction
Functional eyelid abnormality in Down syndrome
Marginal blepharitis

limeters above the medial canthus, a less rigid criteria than that of Shapiro and France (1985).

Other reports have given an incidence of Mongoloid slant between 40 and 90% in Caucasian patients with Down syndrome, and up to 100% in Oriental patients. It is interesting to note that Gifford (1924) reported that in normal patients of Oriental heritage the incidence of significant Mongoloid slant is not greater than that seen in normal patients of Caucasian heritage.

Epicanthal folds are defined as a fold of skin covering all or part of the medial canthal region and conjunctival caruncle, the medial transitional zone between skin, and medial bulbar conjuctiva. Epicanthus was probably first reported formally by Schoen (1828), and was subsequently fully described and classified by Von Ammon and Von Ammon (1831). Epicanthus has been classified in various ways since these initial reports, but probably the most useful classification is that of *simple epicanthus*, where the amount of tissue involved in the fold is the same above and below the medial canthus, *epicanthus tarsalis*, where the fold of skin in the upper lid is larger than that in the lower lid, and *epicanthus inversus*, where the fold in the lower lid is larger than that in the upper lid (see Figure 3.1).

Epicanthal folds are overwhelmingly common in infants of all racial groups, especially among Orientals. Epicanthus is, in fact, so common that it can be thought of as the normal configuration of the infant eyelid. As infants pass through childhood development and growth, the epicanthal folds generally regress, in individuals of European and African race, while they tend to persist in Oriental persons. It is difficult, therefore, to obtain a sense of whether a specific incidence of epicanthal fold is within the normal range or not without reference to the specific age or racial grouping of the study population. Most reports in the literature, particularly those in the older

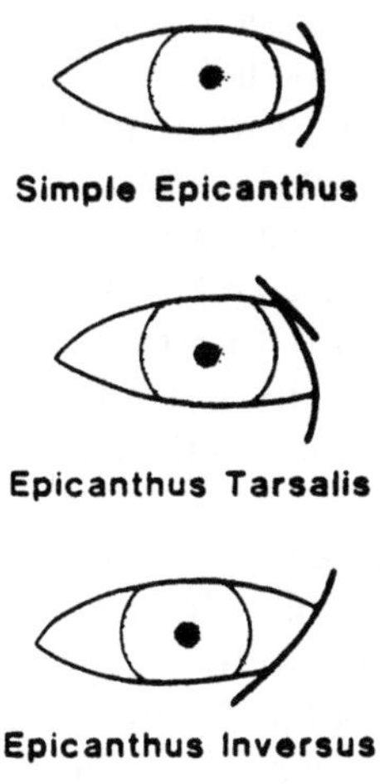

FIGURE 3.1. Epicanthus.

literature, do not control well for age and are misleading. Nevertheless, there is consensus among all investigators writing on the subject that the epicanthal folds are significantly more common in older patients with Down syndrome. Almost all infants with this syndrome do have epicanthal folds; the incidence of significant epicanthal folds decreases with age, though at a much slower rate than in the general population. It appears from reviewing the available literature that 40–50% of patients with Down syndrome, over the age of 10 years, and of European and African extraction, have persistent epicanthal folds, this figure is significantly higher than the 10% incidence in for similarly age- and race-matched control individuals.

The epicanthal fold itself has no functional significance, never being sufficiently broad to obscure any of the nasal visual field. It does give rise to the misapprehension, however, that a very high percentage of patients with these folds have esotropia. This phenomonon is called *pseudostrabismus*, and is responsible for the mistaken impression that many normal young infants, and particularly young children with Down syndrome, have crossed eyes that they later outgrow.

In Down syndrome, the palpebral fissure is generally regarded as having diminished length. Earlier studies suffer from lack of description about how the palpebral fissure length measurements were made, and the more recent research has generally omitted this feature of the eyelid architecture. Specifically, it is not generally noted whether the length of the palpebral fissure is measured from the true medial canthus to the lateral canthus or from the edge of the overlying epicanthal fold. Naturally, if the latter technique were employed, the palpebral fissure would be found to be short in all of those cases having a significantly wide epicanthal fold. If the medial canthus were used as the medical measurement point it would seem that the incidence of short palpebral fissure would be significantly less. In any event, this feature, which is of little functional or cosmetic importance, has not been well studied.

Similarly, hypertelorism (increased interpupillary distance) and telecanthus (increased distance between the medial canthi) have been noted. Again, earlier studies in the literature do not give adequate measurement criteria and do not specify whether the measurements for telecanthus are made from the edges of the epicanthal folds or from the true medial canthi. True hypertelorism is not present in Down syndrome to a significant degree. When measurements are made from true medial canthus to true medial canthus, it is found that telecanthus is also not present to a significant degree. The impression of significant telecanthus is probably produced by measurement from the edges of the medial canthal folds.

The configuration of the upper eyelid margin is worthy of note in patients with Down syndrome. Ordinarily, the margin of the upper eyelid has its highest point approximately one-third the distance from the medial canthus to the lateral canthus. The upward and downward curves of the upper lid are, therefore, asymmetrical, lending a somewhat almond-shaped appearance to the interpalpebral space. In Down syndrome the curve of the upper eyelid margin frequently appears to be much more symmetrical, in that the highest point of curvature is the halfway point between the medial and lateral canthi and the two halves of the curve appear as if they can be superimposed upon one another. This configurational oddity, however, is not unique to Down syndrome, and may be found in up to 10% of the normal Caucasian population.

The anatomical eyelid characteristics of the population with Down syndrome, and without Down syndrome, show many similarities. There is no single pathognomonic feature of eyelid architecture that would allow a diagnosis of Down syndrome. A combination of eyelid physical characteristics in this syndrome however, appears to be instantly recognizable to the trained professional.

Findings and Discussion

With these factors in mind, we did not attempt to tabulate individual eyelid characteristics in the patient population studied at the City of Hope but noted only the presence or absence of those factors. A patient was noted to have typical Down syndrome eyelid configuration if he or she was found to have significant obliquity of the palpebral fissure, combined with the presence of epicanthal folds of any type and a symmetrical curve of the upper eyelid margin (Solomons et al., 1965). Using this criteria, 90% of patients were found to have the typical Down syndrome configuration. Compared to studies previously reported, the author feels that the unusually high incidence of eyelid uniformity among patients was due to the low average age of children in the study. The average age was 4 years, 6 months, with a range in age from 2 months to 20 years. The mean age in the study by Shapiro and France (1985) was 17.4 years, with a range from 7 to 36 years; in the study by Solomons et al. (1965), there is an apparent mean age of approximately 20 years. Although difficult to quantify, the typical eyelid appearance is most prevalent in younger children with Down syndrome, who lose some of their typical features, particularly the epicanthal folds, as they grow older. One patient in the study had no typical eyelid features of Down syndrome; however, prior to the study the patient had reconstructive plastic surgery to eliminate these features.

Down syndrome appears to cause a specific constellation of changes of eyelid morphology that permits an observer to arrive at an overall impression of abnormality, rather than one omnipresent pathognomic change in lid architecture. These changes are all cosmetic in nature, with no visual significance; cosmetic surgical repair can be performed electively.

Marginal Blepharitis

Marginal blepharitis is a condition of the eyelid margins in which the margins become inflamed; in some cases, scaling, exudation, hypervascularity and plugging of the orifices of the Meibomian glands are noted on slit lamp biomicroscopical examination. If unchecked, this inflammation can lead to an irritation of the ocular surface tissues (conjunctivitis) and, in extreme cases, keratitis or corneal inflammation with subsequent corneal scarring. There is increased incidence of marginal blepharitis reported in Down syndrome, with estimates ranging from 2 to 70% (Cullen & Butler, 1963; Shapiro & France, 1985; Sheller & Oster, 1951). This wide disparity of reported incidence may be representative of a lack of precise diagnostic criteria for marginal blepharitis and a lack of uniformity of observational conditions and techniques.

In our study, 13% of the patients had active marginal blepharitis (including eyelid margin scaling, exudation, hypervascularity, and some injection of the adjacent conjunctiva) at the initial evaluation. We emphasize, however, that in all probability this 13% does not represent an overall incidence on a per-patient basis—the patients were examined, in most cases, only once; it is likely that repeated examinations would have revealed more cases of blepharitis. In addition, the younger mean age of the study group should be emphasized, since there is a trend toward higher incidence of marginal blepharitis with increasing age of the patient.

In its early stages, marginal blepharitis may cause ocular itching and irritation. If left untreated this may progress to tearing, significant observable conjunctival inflammation with eyelid crusting, ocular discharge, photophobia, and frank discomfort. Treatment of this condition is relatively simple, consisting of cleansing the eyelid margins with a diluted solution of baby shampoo in warm water (1:5 dilution), followed by application of Bactracin or Erythromycin ophthalmic ointment to the involved areas twice daily. This treatment is generally continued for three to four week until the condition is under control. Since marginal blepharitis tends to be a chronic condition, it is usually beneficial to recommend that the treatment be performed once weekly to prevent recurrence, even after the acute exacerbation has been satisfactorily controlled. When followed, this treatment regime has proven sufficient to control all observed cases. Behavioral disorders may prevent adequate lid hygiene in patients with Down syndrome, but to ignore the problem is to risk the possibility of a chronic condition resulting in discomfort and visual loss Table 3.2.

Anterior Segment Disorders

Cornea

Corneal changes are relatively rare in Down syndrome. In fact, these changes are limited to those of a single entity: keratoconus. This corneal deformity is a condition in which a progressive thinning and stretching of the corneal stromal lamellae develops, accompanied by development of a conical curvature, rather than the generally spherical curvature found in normal individuals. Rarely noted in infancy or early childhood, keratoconus usually becomes

TABLE 3.2. Structural ocular abnormalities in Down syndrome.

Anterior segment	Posterior segment
Cornea	Retina
Keratoconus	Retinal hypopigmentation
Iris	Retinal vascular alterations
Stromal hypoplasia	Increased number of vessels at disk margin
Stromal hypopigmentation	Early-branching arteries
Brushfield nodules	Decreased arterial caliber
Lens	Optic Nerve
Cataract	Optic nerve hypoplasia

more severe as the child grows older. It ultimately may result in an irregularly conical cornea, creating an irregular refraction of the incoming light rays that cannot be resolved to a coherent image on the retina with any known spectacle lens.

In some cases the ectasia and stretching of the cornea become so severe that acute hydrops develops. This situation occurs when the inextensible Descement's membrane (the basement membrane) of the corneal endothelial cells) becomes overstretched and ruptures, allowing aqueous humor from the anterior chamber to rush into the corneal stroma. This excess fluid disrupts the regular lamellar organization of the stroma that is responsible for corneal transparency. Aqueous influx thus results in a central milky opacity of the cornea at the apex of the cone. This opacity may preclude any but the most faulty vision.

The incidence of keratoconus patients with Down syndrome is generally estimated to be 10 % or less Lyle et al., 1972; Shapiro & France, 1985; Sheller & Oster, 1951). The etiology of the conical deformity is unknown. Previous authors have suggested it may be due to repeated trauma caused by eye rubbing in response to chronic blepharitis in these patients or to a basic defect in the corneal collagen matrix. This latter defect has not been found in corneal tissue removed during penetrating keratoplasty in these patients.

Severe cone formation with resultant uncorrectable astigmatism and acute hydrops can be treated with penetrating keratoplasty (corneal transplantation). This procedure is generally quite successful in restoring useful visual acuity, although behavioral disorders leading to accidental or intentional trauma may cause surgical complications in patients with more severe mental retardation. In our study, no patients with keratoconus were found; this is probably related to the preponderance of patients in younger age groups.

Conjunctiva

Structural changes of the conjunctiva have not been reported in Down syndrome. However, patients with Down syndrome frequently have conjunctival vascular injection and inflammation, accompanied by minimal ocular discharge and morning eyelid margin crusting. These changes are usually due to blepharitis of the adjacent eyelids and are termed *blepharoconjunctivitis*. If left untreated, severe blepharoconjunctivitis can lead to corneal inflammation and scarring. Though unproven, this condition has been implicated in the causation of keratoconus through the mechanism of eye rubbing, as previously noted.

Blepharoconjunctivitis, an extension of marginal blepharitis, can be treated in the same manner as marginal blepharitis, with eyelid scrubs followed by topical antibiotic ointment. Treatment in this manner is quite efficacious for providing significant symptomatic relief. Long-term, low-level therapy is frequently required.

Anterior Chamber

Anomalies of the anterior chamber of the eye have not been reported in association with Down syndrome. In the present study, anterior chamber depth appeared similar to that of control subjects.

Iris

Changes in the structure of the iris have been prominently associated with descriptions of Down syndrome since 1902, when Wolfflin described elevated nodules of white or yellow tissue situated in a circular fashion about the periphery of the iris. Microscopically the nodules consisted of condensations of the normal iris stromal connective tissue. Brushfield (1924) subsequently reported these nodules to be characteristic of Down syndrome.

In fact, several structural changes in the iris are positively correlated with this syndrome, including Brushfield spots, hypoplasia of the iris stroma, and decreased iris pigmentation. Brushfield spots, although initially felt to be pathognomonic for Down syndrome, have been found to be present in non-Down syndrome individuals (Donaldson, 1961). The incidence of Brushfield spots has been reported to vary between 13 and 90% in individuals affected with Down syndrome (Eissler & Longenscker, 1962; Lowe, 1949; Lyle et al., 1972; Shapiro & France, 1985; Solomons et al., 1965).

The difference in overall incidence is partially explained by differences in examination technique (direct versus slit lamp examination), the variable distinctness of the spots in different individuals, and the variability in incidence of spotting in different colored irides. The spots are more frequently present in light-colored irides than in dark brown, even on slit lamp biomicroscopy. In fact, several authors have reported a complete absence of Brushfield nodules in brown-eyed Down syndrome individuals (Engler, 1949; Wallis, 1951). This was subsequently found to be incorrect and an incidence of up to 10% in brown-eyed Down syndrome patients is noted (Lowe, 1949). In non–Down syndrome subjects, typical Brushfield spots may be found in 2 to

18%, with light-colored irides again having the high prevalence of Brushfield nodule formation.

Hypoplasia of the iris stroma was first reported by Lowe in 1949, when he found it to be present in 95% of 64 patients. The mid-peripheral zone of the iris is involved, at about the junction of the middle and outer third of the iris, where strands "diminish in number and thickness and become very wavy." As noted by Lowe, thickly pigmented, dark brown irides fail to show this peripheral thinning. In extreme cases, the dark brown posterior pigment epithelium shows through the stroma in light-eyed patients. The incidence of iris stromal hypoplasia has been reported to range between 22 and 94%, Sevineon Freideman and Stamps 1955, while the incidence in non–Down syndrome populations is 9% (Donaldson, 1961). The variability in incidence figures is again probably due to the variable proportion of dark-eyed individuals within the Down syndrome population studied.

Decreased iris pigmentation is probably a reflection of the thinned iris stroma previously noted, since the pigment melanin is located within the stroma. Consistent with this hypothesis is the observation that children with Down syndrome who have very dark-eyed parents, particularly those of Latino or Oriental extraction, do not have noticeably lighter-colored irides than their parents or siblings. This would be expected since their iris stroma is not thin. Down syndrome children of lighter-eyed parents frequently do have lighter-colored irides than their parents and siblings, probably because their iris stroma may be thinner.

In the present study, definite Brushfield spot formation was present in 30% of the patients. This low percentage may have been due to the high proportion of Latino and Oriental subjects within the study, who usually have dark brown irides. Similarly, iris stromal hypoplasia was distinctly present in 10% of the patients studied. In a control group of 100 patients without Down syndrome, 7 had Brushfield spots, and 5 had distinctly hypoplastic peripheral iris stroma.

Lens

The association of cataract, or lens opacity, with Down syndrome has been appreciated since 1910, when Ormond, examining a series of patients with oblique illumination through undilated pupils, described 25 of 42 patients as having dot-like opacities in a lamellar distribution within their lenses. In some patients, additional opacities within the Y-sutures of the lenses and apparent coalescence of the dot opacities into localized masses was noted (Ormond, 1912). Subsequent authors greatly expanded the descriptive material on cataract morphology associated with Down syndrome, and Lowe described the "typical" Down syndrome cataract in 1949 (Brushfield, 1924; Lowe, 1949; Van der Scheer, 1927).

Lowe's description emphasized "flake-like" opacities in a circular distribution within the midperiphery of the lens, probably within the cortex. The flakes are described and drawn as ranging in size up to one-quarter of a millimeter in diameter, but very thin; so thin, in fact, that they are frequently invisible on direct illumination, showing up even the under microscope only under oblique or retro-illumination. The flakes are described as variable in color, ranging from white to blue, with even a few that are light brown. There appears to be a tendency toward progression or increase in opacification, since several of the authors note that opacities are few or absent in young patients and become more frequent as the population ages.

As with other ocular abnormalities previously discussed, the reported incidence is highly variable, ranging from 12 to 46%. Again, this variability is probably due to variation in methods of examination, which range from direct visualization and illumination through the use of the direct ophthalmoscope and retro-illumination ("red reflex") through dilated or undilated pupils, to the use of the slip lamp biomicroscope, the most accurate method. To compound the difficulty in understanding the significance of cataract formation in these patients, many authors do not state whether or not the opacities are visually significant. Some do mention visual significance but do not provide any quantification of acuity loss. It must be recalled, however, that visual acuity data are frequently difficult to obtain in patients with Down syndrome because of their diminished mental capacity.

In general, only cataracts that impinge on the central (visual) axis of the lens are visually debilitating. The "typical" early Down syndrome cataract, frequently peripheral in location, is probably of little or no visual significance. Similarly, sutural opacities are rarely visually inhibitory. Thus, in children with this syndrome, a cataract is rarely the cause of significant visual disability. As patients grow older, however, their "flakes" become more numerous and central and a measurable loss of visual acuity may occur.

In the present study, 42% of patients were found to have some lenticular opacities, including minor ones. This unusually high percentage, despite the young average age of our patients (4 years, 6 months), was documented by the use of a combination of examination techniques including slit lamp examination and direct ophthalmoscopy with retro-illumination, both tests performed after pupillary dilation. Visually significant lens opacities, however, were much less common; only 8% of our patients (12 patients) had a visual acuity loss of greater than two lines of acuity using Allen symbol testing for acuity. Among these patients, seven had flake-like opacities, four had sheet-like cortical cataracts, and one had a combined anterior polar and posterior subcapsular cataract. Two of the patients with flake cataract had documented progression of the cataract centrally over a two-year time span, with a further decrease in visual acuity.

Cataracts are treated, at present, by surgical removal of the opacified lens, followed by replacement of the now-absent optical power of the missing lens with an intraocular lens implant, a contact lens, or spectacles. In former times, cataract surgery was relatively crude and frequently likely to engender complications, especially in subjects unable to cooperate postoperatively with a regime of bed rest or other limited activity. The advent of modern surgical techniques for cataract removal, including aspiration or suction/cutting through small incisions, followed by wound repair with ultrafine, strong microsurgical sutures, as well as advances in safety of general anesthesia, has made cataract removal a practical therapy for patients with Down syndrome, and one that should be readily employed once visually significant cataracts are present. Of the available optical replacement techniques, intraocular lens implantation is to be preferred, since it requires the least postoperative cooperation for visual rehabilitation.

Lowe remarked in 1949, "As the older patients require relatively little vision for their interests, extremely few of them need any surgical intervention." This view, and others similarly expressed in the past, reflect undue pessimism about both the mental capacity and likelihood of surgical success in these patients. Fortunately, our surgical techniques have advanced sufficiently to visually rehabilitate almost all patients with debilitating cataract, and we do not need to rationalize our lack of surgical success by assuming a diminished need for sensory contact with the outside world in these patients. Successful cataract surgery has produced a gratifyingly positive emotional and functional response in patients with Down syndrome.

Vitreous—no significant abnormalities of vitreous structure or composition have been found in association with Down syndrome.

Posterior Segment

In contrast to the large number of papers describing the various anterior segment and adenexal abnormalities associated with Down syndrome, there is a striking paucity of description of posterior segment anomalies. This lack of material in the literature could lead one to conclude that the various structures within the ocular fundus were rarely affected by Down syndrome, but this conclusion would be erroneous. In fact, structural changes are quite frequent in certain posterior structures, although this unsuspected frequency and the characteristics of two disorders are reported herein for the first time.

It would appear that the scarcity of mention of posterior segment disorders in early literature was related to inadequate examination technique rather than lack of findings. Prior to World War II, fundoscopic examination was carried out with a *direct* ophthalmoscope. This instrument is notoriously difficult to use in an uncooperative subject because of the relatively narrow field of view afforded, necessitating observation of many separate small fields with a subsequent "integration" of these discrete areas into a coherent overall picture within the mind of the observer. Although small details can be appreciated with this method, one tends to lose some aspects of the overall pattern; one "can't see the forest for the trees." Additionally, the peripheral fundus cannot be visualized at all with a direct ophthalmoscope.

After World War II the *indirect* ophthalmoscope was introduced and popularized. Although this instrument has the disadvantages of requiring pupillary dilation for examination and providing less magnification than the direct ophthalmoscope, its wide-angle view of about 25 degrees versus about 4 degrees for the direct ophthalmoscope renders it a superb instrument for appreciation of overall fundus architectural patterns. The retina can easily be examined all the way to the equator, even in uncooperative subjects, and with the addition the technique of scleral depression the entire retina to the ora serrata can be examined.

Despite the advantage in instrumentation, relatively few papers on fundus architecture in Down syndrome have appeared in recent years. This may reflect the inability of any medical practitioners except ophthalmologists to use the indirect ophthalmoscope, and a pervasive belief among ophthalmologists that patients with Down syndrome are difficult to examine. This belief is patently false. Down syndrome patients, like pediatric patients in general, can usually be examined with indirect ophthalmoscopy if they are treated in a nonthreatening manner, examined quickly, and if their attention is diverted elsewhere during the examination by animated fixation toys, movies, videotapes, etc. A patient rarely requires light sedation if a detailed examination is required.

Retina

Retinal anomalies have only rarely been reported in Down syndrome. Mention has been made within the context of general reviews of the subject or during reports on other subjects of neuro-retinitis (Oliver, 1891; Skeller & Oster, 1951), peripapillary crescents and pigmented ares, colobomata, and choroidal breaks (Gannon & Schimek, 1977). However, all of these findings may simply represent the coincidental occurrence of rare ocular anomalies in a relatively common disorder like Down syndrome.

Ahmad and Pruett (1976) have provided a prospective survey of the fundi of 32 patients with Down syndrome. All of the patients were examined by indirect ophthalmoscopy with scleral depression. Minimal choroidal vascular "sclerosis" was found in all patients over 20 years of age. Three patients had temporary whitening of choroidal vessels, three had peripheral localized patches of choroidal atrophy, and four had hyperpigmented peripheral spots. Peripheral cystoid degeneration along the ora serrata was found in all 30 eyes examined with scleral depression. The maculae showed no abnormalities. It must be emphasized that none of the preceding lesions resulted in any visual loss.

Interestingly, all patients examined, irrespective of skin and iris pigmentation, exhibited a paucity of fundus pigmentation similar to that noted in blond individuals. This may be like the decreased pigmentation previously mentioned in the irides of patients with Down syndrome.

In the present study, a similar paucity of fundus pigmentation was noted in most of the patients, except for those with dark-pigmented skin and irides.

This lack of pigmentation is difficult to quantify on the basis of examination alone and fundus photography was not routinely performed.

Ahmad and Pruett (1976) also present case reports of six patients with retinal detachment. It must be emphasized that these patients were not found in the course of the routine survey of the 32 patients previously mentioned—they were patients known to the authors as having retinal detachment and Down syndrome. The true incidence of retinal detachment in this syndrome cannot be estimated from this data. Undoubtedly the incidence is quite low, in view of the rarity of reports in the literature. Ahmad and Pruett (1976) emphasize the relation of datachment to trauma; peripheral facial nerve paralysis, head banging, violent rubbing of the eyes, corneal abrasion, hyphema, angle recession, subluxation, and retinal dialysis, all signs of trauma, were observed in these patients.

Retinal Vasculature

As there was no mention in the literature before 1973, the retinal blood vessels were felt to be either normal or unremarkable by the reviewers of ophthalmic changes in the patient with Down syndrome. Williams et al., (1973) reviewed the fundi of 50 institutionalized Down patients and compared them to 50 age- and sex-matched controls. These authors were hopeful that the changes would be "helpful in the diagnosis of Mongolism." Their findings consisted of an increased number of retinal blood vessels crossing the margins of the optic nerve head. Forty-four of 50 mongoloid patients (88%) had 16 or more vessels crossing the disk margins, while only 8 of 50 (16%) normal controls had 16 or more vessels in the same area. No individual with Down syndrome had fewer than 13 vessels, but 16 of 50 (32%) control patients had fewer than 13 vessels crossing the disk margin. Seventeen of 50 patients had more than 18 disk vessels (34%), while only one control (2%) had more than 18. These differences were statistically significant ($p < 0.01$).

In addition to the quantitative differences observed, Williams et al. (1973) comment on the pattern of distribution of fundus vessels, which appeared different from normal in Down syndrome patients. In nonsyndrome patients, the vessels of the fundus appear to arch temporally around the macular region, branching some distance away from the disk. In patients with this syndrome, the vessels appear to radiate (like spokes) directly from the disk with few branchings. Williams et al. (1973) comment that the "spoke" pattern appears to be due to the result of early bifurcation of vessels before they cross the optic disk margin. In fact, since bifurcation on the disk surface is almost never seen in patients with Down syndrome (personal data), the bifurcations must have occurred posterior to the surface of the disk, between that area and the area that lies approximately 8 to 12 millimeters posterior to the globe, where the central retinal artery and vein enter the optic nerve and bifurcate initially as they pass forward to the lamina cribrosa (Last, 1968).

TABLE 3.3. Study of retinal vessels in Down syndrome.

	N	%	N	%
	> 16 vessels[a]		> 18 vessels[b]	
DS; 150 patients (300 eyes)	112	75	78	52
Non-DS/control; 100 patients (200 eyes)	9	9	2	2

[a]Greater than 16 vessels at disk margin.
[b]Greater than 18 vessels at disk margin.
N = Numbers of *patients* found with this condition.

With these previous findings in mind, the retinal blood vessels of the 150 patients (300 eyes) in the present study were examined carefully and compared to those of 100 non–Down syndrome controls (200 eyes) with a view to confirming and extending the findings of Williams et al. (1973). In this way it was hoped that a highly characteristic ophthalmic sign of Down syndrome could be elucidated. Our data showed that 75% of the eyes examined showed greater than 16 vessels at the disk margin in the group having Down syndrome, while 9% of the control patients had similar numbers of vessels at the disk margin (see Table 3). In the eyes of persons with Down syndrome, 52% of patients had more than 18 vessels at the disk margin. Two control patient eyes (from the same patient) had similar findings. These data appeared to confirm those of Williams et al. (1973). Our observations also agreed with regard to the overall architecture of the retinal vasculature: the vessels in the Down syndrome patient proceed outward from the disk in a more direct, spoke-like, less curvilinear fashion that those of normal controls.

Close study of the vascular pattern of the fundus in these patients with Down syndrome has permitted two additional characteristics of the fundus vascularization to be delineated. First, the increase in number of Down syndrome vessels at the disk margin appears to be largely due to an increase in the number of *arteries* present. The veins are *not* increased in number when compared to those of the controls using statistical methods. Indeed, it often appears ophthalmoscopically that the arteries are doubled, with a pair of arteries heading together in the same general direction as one vein from the region of the posterior pole. Additionally, the caliber of the arteries appears diminished when compared to the arteries of control subjects and when compared to the veins in the same patient, as if the same blood flow as in normals were being carried in more arteries of smaller diameter, which drain into fewer, larger veins of more normal caliber. Measurement of actual vascular caliber could not be carried out within the limits of the present study, but the differences from normal do appear striking to this observer, as if there were at least one-third diminution of arterial caliber.

The vascular patterns of the fundus allows one to confidently predict whether a patient does or does not have Down syndrome. Subsequent to the performance of this study, I examined over 2000 fundi in unselected patients under 18 years of age and I was unable to find a single non–Down syndrome

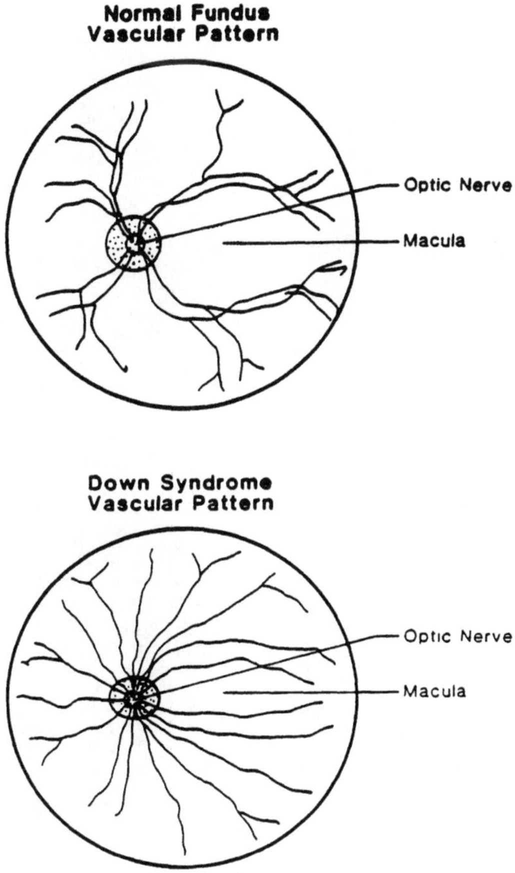

FIGURE 3.2. Fundus vascular pattern in Down syndrome, diagrammatic representations.

patient who combines the characteristic picture of increased number and decreased caliber of arteries within the typical spoke-like directional pattern. Additionally, using this combination of signs I have been able to correctly predict the presence of Down syndrome in 11 newborn infants prior to diagnosis by their attending pediatrician or confirmation by chromosome analysis. No false diagnoses have been made by this method. I have not yet studied whether or not the different chromosomal patterns of Down syndrome result in different vascular patterns, but at present this does not seem to be the case. Of some interest is the finding that the retinal vascular changes associated with Down syndrome are present at birth.

Thus our present study demonstrates the presence of a characteristic fundus vascular architecture in this syndrome. This characteristic appearance may be as typical of Down syndrome as facial appearance or dermatoglyphic pattern.

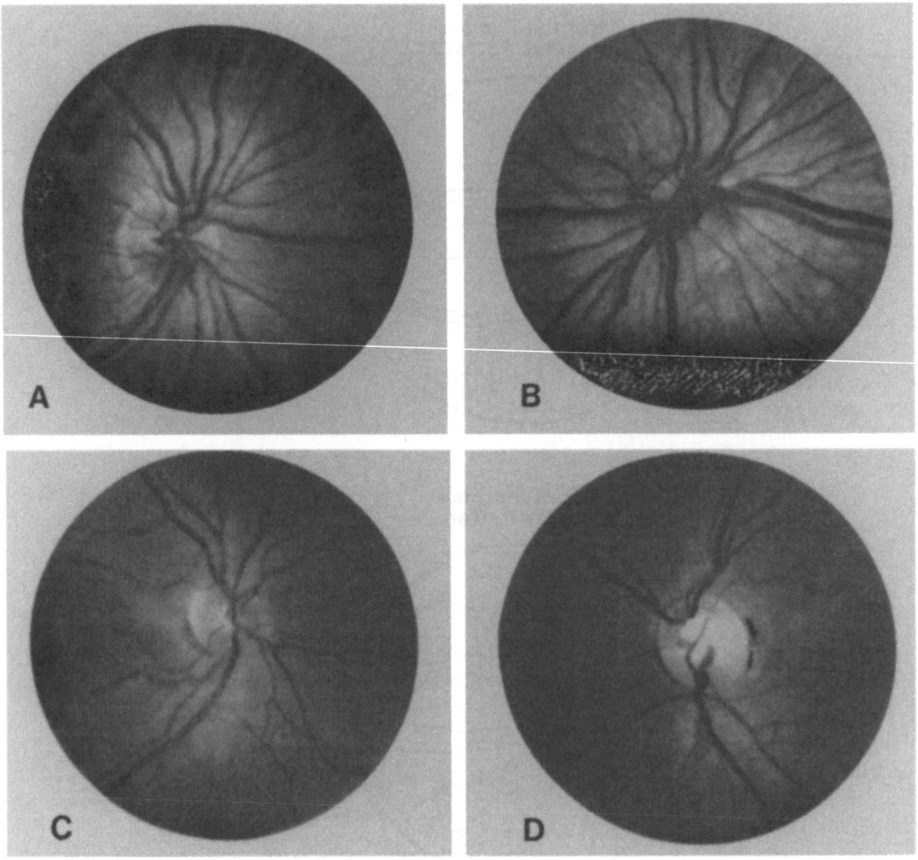

FIGURE 3.3A. Fundus of 20 year-old female with Down syndrome with 21 vessels crossing margin of the optic nerve head. A spoke-like pattern of vessels is present.

FIGURE 3.3B. Fundus of 19-year-old male with Down syndrome with 20 vessels crossing margin of the optic nerve head. A spoke-like pattern of vessels is present.

FIGURE 3.3C. Fundus of 17-year-old male control with 12 vessels crossing margin of the optic nerve head. A nonlinear, branching pattern of vessels is present.

FIGURE 3.3D. Fundus of an 18-year-old female control with 10 vessels crossing margin of the optic nerve head. A nonlinear, branching pattern of vessels is present.

Figures 3.3A–3.3D reprinted with permission from: Williams, E.T., McCormick, A.Q., Tischler, B.(1973). Retinal vessels in Down's syndrome, *Archives of Ophthalmology, 89*, 269–271.

Optic Nerve

Except for one isolated case report discussing one patient, optic nerve anomalies have not been reported in association with Down syndrome. In that report, Awan (1977) presents a case of "ganglionic neuroretinal hypoplasia" (hypoplasia of the optic nerve head). This one-year-old female also was noted to have esotropia, diminished fixation with one eye, pendular nystagmus, and impatency of the nasolacrimal ducts with epiphora since birth. During the course of a nasolacrimal duct probing for the latter problem, an examination including ophthalmoscopy was performed under anesthesia, this examination showed a normal right fundus with typical findings of optic nerve hypoplasia in the left eye (Awan, 1977). The author recommended "an active search for these ocular changes...in cases of Down syndrome." Despite this advice, given in 1977, no further cases have been reported.

Optic nerve hypoplasia is a congenital anomaly of the optic nerve in which a diminished number of axons are present in the involved nerve when compared to the normal. The condition is nonprogressive, representing a true absence of fibers at birth rather than an acquired optic atrophy. The involved nerve heads are variable in appearance, ranging from nearly total aplasia to subtle segmental deficits. The most characteristic appearance is that of the "double ring" sign, which refers to the diminished optic nerve head, usually more intensely pink than usual with little or no cup, and surrounded by a yellow or white ring, in turn surrounded by a hyperpigmented choroidal ring. To the untrained observer, the concentric rings give the superficial appearance of a normal disk surrounded by a peripapillary hyperpigmented ring and halo, a not uncommon anatomical situation. Close inspection reveals that the optic nerve tissue is actually only the intensely pink central tissue, with the pale area surrounding it representing only scleral and glial tissue (Lambert et al., 1987).

Visual acuity is quite variable in cases of optic nerve hypoplasia. The appearance of the disk is not necessarily a good predictor of ultimate visual acuity since the missing fibers might be from peripheral retina rather than the fovea (Smith, 1980).

While optic nerve hypoplasia was initially considered to be an isolated anomaly, this is now known to be untrue in many instances. Peterson and Walton (1977) described 17 patients with optic nerve hypoplasia and good visual acuity, all of whom were children of diabetic mothers. Since that time it has also been reported in median facial cleft syndrome, Duane syndrome, Klippel-Trenaunay-Weber syndrome, Goldenhar-Glotz-Gorlin syndrome, chondrodysplasia punctata, Meckel syndrome, orbital Apert syndrome, hypertelorism, hemifacial atrophy, blepharophimosis syndrome, and de Morsier syndrome (septo-optic dysplasia). Neurological associations include anencephaly, porencephaly, cerebral atrophy, hydroancephaly, and encephalocele (Lambert et al., 1987).

In the series of patients reported here, an unexpectedly high incidence of optic nerve hypoplasia was noted. Sixteen patients with Down syndrome

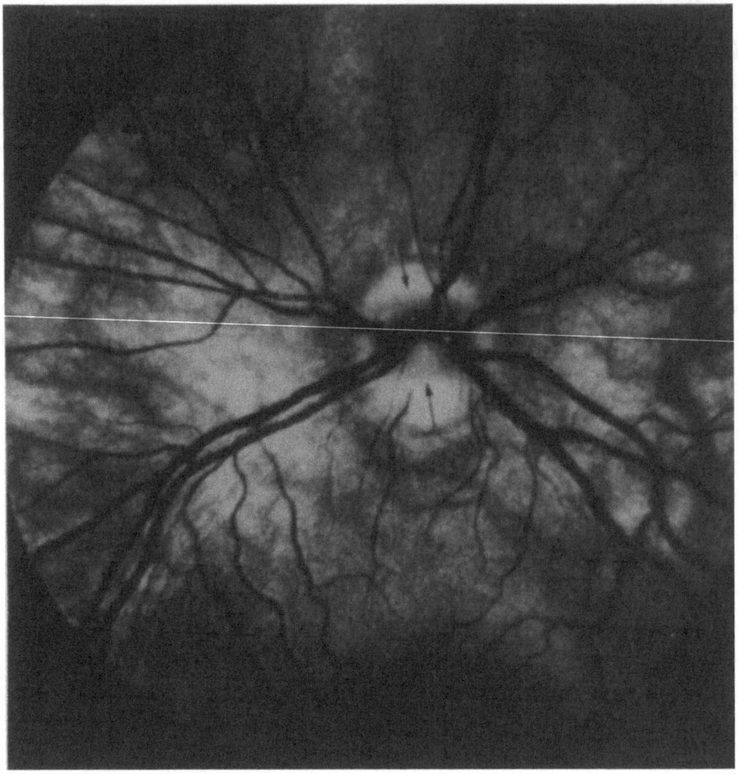

FIGURE 3.4. Optic nerve hypoplasia. Reprinted with permission from: Lambert, S.R., Hoyt, C.S., Narahara, M.H. (1987). Optic nerve hypoplasia. *Survey of Ophthalmology, 32* (1) 1–9.

(10.1% of those examined) had optic nerve hypoplasia documented by the presence of a typical double ring sign. In 14 of the 16 patients the hypoplasia was bilateral; in two cases it was unilateral. None of the 16 patients had significant nystagmus, but three patients had esotropia. In the series of 100 control patients, no patient had ophthalmoscopic findings of optic nerve hypoplasia.

In view of this striking incidence, one must include optic nerve hypoplasia as one of the expected ocular anomalies of Down syndrome. Its presence should be suspected and diligently searched for in all Down syndrome patients. It is of note that in no case within this series did the optic nerve hypoplasia appear to cause serious visual loss. Most of the patients were too young and uncooperative for standard Snellen visual acuity testing, but in the six patients in whom Allen symbol testing could be accomplished, 12 eyes had a visual acuity of not less than 15/30 (20/40 in Snellen terms). One should not automatically ascribe serious visual loss to optic nerve hypoplasia when present; Other causes, like significant refractive error and/or amblyopia, should be carefully searched for and corrected when found, even in an eye with a hypoplastic nerve head.

Nystagmus

Nystagmus consists of rhythmic oscillations or tremor-like movements of the eyes (Walsh & Hoyt, 1969). The condition may be unilateral or, more commonly, bilateral. Nystagmus may be pendular (movement in each direction is of the same velocity), jerk-type (slow movement in one direction coupled with a rapid corrective movement in the opposite direction), rotary, or mixed. True nystagmus must be distinguished from pseudonystagmus or endpoint nystagmus, in which the eyes shake at an extreme of lateral or vertical range. This is likened to the limb shaking that occurs on maximal muscular effort. In general, pendular nystagmus is sensory in origin. It is associated with severe visual loss, as in cases of infantile cataract or extreme refractive error. Other forms of nystagmus, often wrongly called motor nystagmus, are probably related to disordered central nervous system processing of ocular positional responses, but their mechanism has not been precisely elucidated.

Nystagmus was first reported in Down syndrome by Sutherland (1989). it has not been found to be a prominent feature, for it is usually present in fewer than 20% of all cases (Eissler & Longenecker, 1962; Gannon & Schimek, 1977; Lowe, 1949; Lyle et al., 1972; Shapiro & France, 1985; Skeller & Oster, 1951). Most of these cases were due to defects in visual acuity, and most authors have concluded that Down syndrome does not include a specific or characteristic defect of oculomotor control.

In our present study, nystagmus was present in 15 cases (10%). Fourteen of these patients had jerk-type nystagmus, and one had rotary nystagmus. No cases of pendular nystagmus were noted. One case of nystagmus appeared in the setting of a typical case of spasms nutans with head nodding. Five cases were associated with strabismus (Table 3.4). Interestingly, in no case was nystagmus associated with the optic nerve hypoplasia previously described in this chapter. It might be expected that severe hypoplasia of the optic nerve would produce pendular nystagmus.

Strabismus

Strabismus may be defined as a deviation of the visual axis of the eyes; an attempt on the part of the subject to gaze at an object does not result in the image of that object falling simultaneously on the fovea of each eye. This deviation maybe either intermittent or constant, and its direction may be either inward (esotropia), outward (exotropia), upward (hypertropia), or a combination of these. Approximately 1 to 2% of the general population has strabismus in some form.

TABLE 3.4. Abnormalities of ocular alignment in Down syndrome.

Abnormality	Reported incidence[a] (%)	Current study incidence: Number of patients	(%)
Strabismus	*32–44*	*55*	*37*
Esotropia	30–44	*50*	34
Accommodative	15		5
Nonaccommodative	19		30
Exotropia	0–6	*5*	3
A-pattern	3		2
V-pattern	2		3
Oblique muscle dys.	1		5
Nystagmus		*15*	10
Horizontal jerk-type	5–15		10
Rotary type	5		1

[a]Summary of incidence figures (when available) in all papers reviewed.

In most cases, the precise etiology of strabismus is unknown. Although in a small percentage of cases a single extraocular muscle or cranial nerve supplying that muscle can be shown to be paralyzed or weakened, this is not true in the majority of cases. It seems that the affected individual's central coordination or the interplay of sensory input and motor effect is faulty; that is, in most cases strabismus may be the result of a subtle brain defect. Some evidence for this assumption can be gleaned from the observation that strabismus is far more common among children with any form of brain damage that in the general population.

In some cases, loss of input from one eye may lead to strabismus, as in the presence of a dense unilateral cataract or corneal opacity or, analogously, the presence unilaterally of a large refractive error. In these cases the strabismus is termed "secondary."

The inability to achieve simultaneous bifoveal fixation (the presence of strabismus) leads to loss of single binocular vision. In an adult the development of strabismus usually leads to double vision or diplopia; this is not so in children, especially infants and young children. Various sensory adaptations occur in younger children that enable them to escape diplopia. A complete discussion of these sensory adaptations is beyond the scope of this chapter, but it is sufficient to say that all rely to some degree on the ability of the individual to suppress, temporarily or permanently, the sensory input from one of the two foveas.

From the earliest recognition of Down syndrome, strabismus has been recognized as an important constituent. Brushfield (1924) reported, "Every mongol examined has exhibited this [strabismus] in a more or less degree without exception; it was a constant symptom in my cases." This assertion is, however, probably a gross overstatment due to the author's failure to distinguish between true esotropia and pseudoestropia, the esotropic appearance caused in a subject by the presence of epicanthal folds and a wide, flat nasal bridge, such as many infants and Orientals possess. Since these are common facial features in Down syndrome, it is easy to see why one might think all victims of this syndrome have strabismus.

The true incidence of the strabismus is somewhat less, though still quite substantial when compared to the general population. Lowe (1949) noted constant strabismus in 33%; Sheller and Oster (1951) in 34%; Shapiro and France (1985) in 43%; Eissler and Longencker (1962) in 44%; and Hiles, Hoyme, and McFarlane (1974) in 34% in a retrospective study devoted exclusively to Down syndrome and strabismus. Interestingly, all the authors report an overwhelming propensity toward esotropia among the strabismus; exotropia and hypertropia (unassociated with estropia) were quite rare. This is perhaps not so surprising when one is made aware of the preponderance of esotropia among early onset strabismus (birth to 6 months) in the general population. Strabismus in patients with Down syndrome is usually of early onset.

Hiles et al. (1974) indicate that the nature of the strabismus in Down syndrome is not fundamentally different from that in the general population and that the same treatment modalities for strabismus can be applied to these patients as to non–Down syndrome patients. If left untreated, strabismus may result in the loss of binocular fusion, binocular depth perception, and a loss of vision in one eye when that eye is subjected to continuous suppression. Appropriate treatment modalities for ocular misalignment include glasses for all significant refractive errors, especially hyperopia in esotropes, prisms (rarely), and surgery.

In the present study, 55 patients were found to have strabismus (37%). Of this number, 50 were esotropes and 5 exotropes (Table 3.4). This preponderence of esotropia was consistent with all other case reports. No primary hypertropias were found.

Of the 50 patients with exotropia, 8 had purely accommodative exotropia that was satisfactorily controlled with glasses. The remainder were all either partially accommodative or nonaccommodative. Three patients had significant V-patterns with greatest esotropia in down gaze, while two patients had A-patterns with greatest esotropia in upgaze. In all 5 cases the pattern was associated with marked oblique overaction, inferior oblique overaction with V-patterns, and superior oblique overaction with A-patterns. This is consistent with the association of A- and V-patterns with oblique muscle dysfunction in strabismus in patients without Down syndrome (Figures 3.2, 3.3).

Refractive Error

Refractive error may be defined as the condition that results when, with accommodation relaxed, parallel light rays are not brought to a discrete single point focus on the retina by the optical refracting surfaces of the involved eye. In effect, almost all eyes have some minimal degree of theoretical refractive error. However, when appreciable image degradation is caused by refractive error, we call that refractive error significant. Hyperopic refractive errors (far-sightedness) can be partially compensated for by the facility of accommodation, which in the human eye can be achieved by contraction of the ciliary muscle to relax the zonules that suspend the lens in its proper position, allowing it to thicken along the visual axis thus increasing its overall net refractive index. No such compensatory ability exists for myopia (near-sightedness) or astigmatism, so that even small amounts of these two conditions result in some degree of image degradation. Therefore, a smaller amount of myopia and astigmatism than hyperopia is required to create a significant refractive error.

Refractive errors can be most conveniently treated in patients with Down syndrome, as with most other pediatric patients, with spectacles. It should be noted that the prescription for spectacles for these or any other patients does not require the active cooperation of the patient; rather, the spectacles may be given on the basis of a prescription derived from a cycloplegic retinoscopy with the usual subjective refinement performed in the technique used by ophthalmologists and optometrists on cooperative adult and older pediatric patients. In experienced hands, cycloplegic retinoscopy should result in an error in the final prescription of no greater than 5 to 10% of optical power and axis. Retinoscopy can be performed on almost all subjects with clear corneas, lenses, and vitreous, except for those who are violently combative. In those cases, light sedation with, for example, chloral hydrate given orally, can be used. There is no reason why any patient with Down syndrome could not at least be tried in the appropriate spectacles if needed.

While most refractive errors can also be corrected with contact lenses, the difficulty in adequately cleansing and caring for these lenses in uncooperative subjects makes these devices less useful for Down syndrome patients; in some instances, however, they have been used successfully. Their use is mandatory in some cases of unilateral congenital cataracts.

Myopia

Myopia, or near-sightedness, is the condition that results when parallel rays of light are brought to a point focus at some finite distance anterior to the fovea rather than on the foveal retina. The reported incidence of significant myopia in the general population has been somewhat variable in past studies. Sorsby et al., (1960) found that approximately 2% of men were more myopic than −4.00 diopters and that 9% of men were myopic to less than −4.00 diopters. Most authors have found a normal distribution of refractive errors surrounding the emmetropic, or zero refractive point.

In the present study, 12% of patients had myopia of more than −2.00 diopters, and 6 patients (4%) had myopia of worse than −6.00 diopters. The greatest degree of myopia noted was −21.00 diopters. These incidence figures are probably not significantly different from those of the general population, and are not in accord with previous assertions that the incidence of myopia is higher in patients with Down syndrome than in patients without.

Myopia is most appropriately treated in patients with Down syndrome through the use of spectacles. Contact lenses are theoretically possible in these patients, but lack of adequate cooperation and motivation frequently renders their use less than ideal. Since an adequate diagnostic refraction can be carried out with cycloplegic retinoscopy on even uncooperative subjects, glasses can at least be tried on all subjects.

Hyperopia

Hyperopia, or far-sightedness, is present when the point image of parallel rays of light is a virtual image at some finite distance posterior to the retina. This occurs when the refractive media of the eye does not cause sufficient convergence of the parallel rays to allow them to come to a point focus on the retina. In younger patients, hyperopia of moderate or low degrees is a less severe problem than myopia, since it can be overcome by accommodation, large reserves of which are present in younger persons. However, as a subject advances toward middle age the facility of accommodation is lost and hyperopia causes an equal visual degradation to corresponding amounts of myopia. In general, lower degrees of hyperopia (up to 2.00 diopters) do not require any correction during childhood. Hyperopia (at greater than +3.00 diopters) may cause some fatigue of the accommodative mechanism, particularly in older children, adolescents, and adults, and should be corrected with spectacles, particularly when the subject engages in prolonged periods of near-task attention.

The reported incidence of significant hyperopia in the general population depends on the criteria used for reporting and is somewhat variable. Sorsby et al. (1960) report that 75% of men had refractive states between zero and +2.00 diopters of hyperopia, and that 14% of men had hyperopia of greater than 2.00 diopters. It should be noted that all authors report that hyperopia (to a modest degree) is a normal feature of childhood, with the average refraction of one- to two-year-old children falling at about the +2.00-diopter hyperopia range. The degree of hyperopia decreased progressively during childhood and early adolescence.

In the present study 18% of patients refracted had greater than +3.00 diopters of hyperopia. More than half of these patients were esotropic, showing the strong relationship between higher degrees of hyperopia and the development accommodative esotropia. The highest degree of hyperopia noted was +9.00 diopters.

Astigmatism

Astigmatism is a more difficult refractive condition to understand conceptually than either myopia or hyperopia. In astigmatism the resultant refraction of light rays in all meridia is not equal. This results in having parallel rays of light never being brought to a point focus. Most instances of astigmatism in humans are regular; the refractive curves of the eye can be described by formuli such that there is a meridian of least power at 90 degrees to a meridian of greatest power. The net result of the presence of regular astigmatism is the production of an image that is somewhat blurred and distorted, the degree of distortion being proportional to the degree of astigmatism. Despite the conceptual difficulty in understanding astigmatism, the correction is as straightforward when it is regular as the correction of the other two major refractive errors, myopia and hyperopia, namely, the provision of appropriate spectacle lenses. In these cases the spectacle lenses are ground in such a way that they have curves that are essentially opposite in relative weakness and strength to those of the eye to be corrected. The resultant optical combination gives one a spherical result with a point image focused on the foveal area of the retina.

Astigmatism is defined not only by power, but also by the meridian along which that power is exerted. Thus, one commonly speaks of a certain amount of astigmatism at a given axis. In some conventions the axis of greatest power is noted, while in others the axis of least power is noted. It is of some interest that the effect of astigmatism on degradation of visual clarity appears to be least when the axis of astigmatism is at or near the 90-degree or vertical meridian. this angle of astigmatism is called "with the rule" because it is the axis at which the majority of astigmatism occurs in the general population. "Against the rule" astigmatism plus axis is horizontal (along the 180-degree meridian). Oblique astigmatism occurs at axes away from either with the rule or against the rule astigmatism.

Astigmatism may be present in eyes tht are significantly hyperopic or myopic, creating a compound refractive error. These refractive errors may be easily corrected using lenses that combine both spherical and additional meridional power to neutralize both the spherical and astigmatic refractive errors.

The incidence of astigmatism greater than 2.00 diopters in the general population is approximately 15% (Sorsby et al., 1960). In the present study, 35% of patients had astigmatic refractive errors of greater than 2.00 diopters. This is about twice that of the general population. Astigmatism thus seems to be the most characteristic refractive error of Down syndrome. As with other refractive errors, astigmatism is most appropriately corrected in Down syndrome patients by prescription of spectacles.

As interesting correlation has been found in the data from the patient population from the City of Hope betwen the presence of Down syndrome and the direction of the axis of astigmatism. In Figure 3.5, it can be seen that the astigmatic axis of an eye can range from horizontal (0 degrees) to vertical (90 degrees), and back to horizontal (180 degrees). In general, astigmatism plus axes in the general population are most frequently grouped around the 90-degree axis and the 180-degree axis, with the former group somewhat more common. Since astigmatism appears to be evenly distributed on either side of

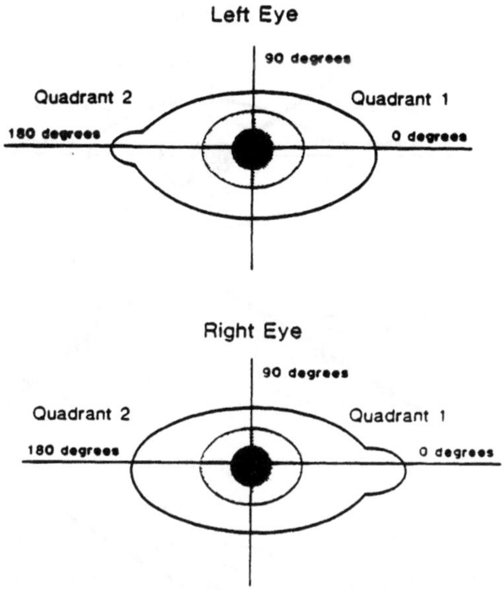

FIGURE 3.5. Axes of astigmatism.

the 90-degree axis, a large population survey reveals an equal number of right eyes with plus axes in quadrant one as in quadrant two (Figure 3.5), and the same is true of left eyes.

In the current study of Down syndrome patient refractive errors, the distribution of axes does not appear to be random. In the right eyes, 90% of the axes of astigmatism for each right eye fall within quadrant one, while for left eyes, 90% of axes fall within quadrant two; an arrangement like the limbs of a capital letter "A" when the patient is viewed from in front.

It might be supposed that this lack of random distribution of axes of astigmatism could be the result of some structural characteristic or defect of the eye symptomatic of Down syndrome. No direct data is present in this study to confirm this supposition. Robb (1977) has reported that the presence of a giant eyelid hemangioma results in the formation of astigmatism with plus axis directed toward the center of the lesion. More recently other authors have confirmed this observation and the theory has arisen that astigmatism may be the product of directional pressure exerted on the growing eye by various eyelid factors like tumors, ptosis, etc. Since the eyelid configuration of Down syndrome is almost uniformly abnormal, it is reasonable to postulate that this results in a fairly uniform deviation of Down syndrome astigmatism from normal distribution. Unfortunately, no data are available to directly confirm this suppostion.

The striking localization of the axis of astigmatism in Down syndrome has some practical application in retinoscopy of these patients. Since they are

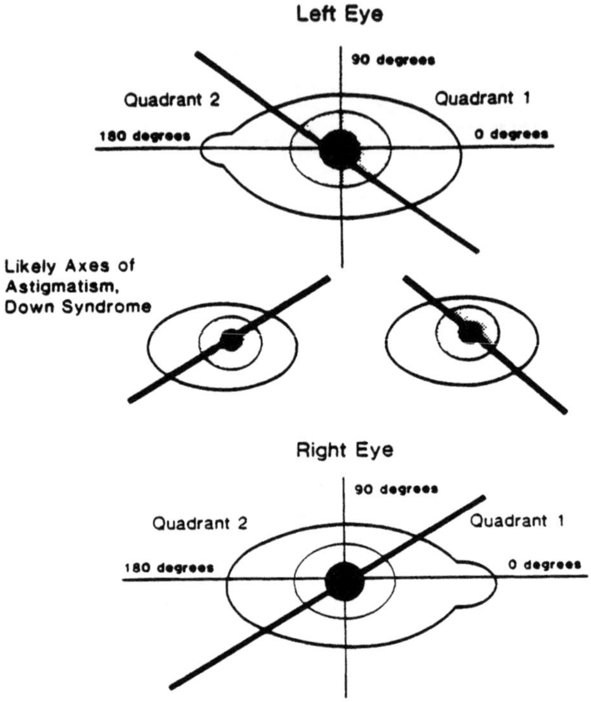

FIGURE 3.6. Axes of astigmatism in Down syndrome.

frequently minimally cooperative, speed in performing retinoscopy is valuable and any information that helps to locate the axis of astigmatism quickly is useful. The author feels this trend of axis location is so consistent that when retinoscoping a patient with Down syndrome, the area around 75 degrees should be checked first in the right eye, and the area around 105 degrees in the left eye, for a plus axis of astigmatism. Similarly, one must view with suspicion retinoscopic results in which the axis of astigmatism for the right eye is between 90 and 180 degrees, and the axis for the left eye is between zero and 90 degrees.

Summary

Uncorrectable visual loss has often been regarded, particularly in the early literature, as a frequent consequence of Down syndrome. Lowe (1949), in his exhaustive review of the subject, reported that the best visual acuity he could obtain from any patient with this syndrome was 20/40 in the better eye, with the implication that many patients were worse. However, careful reading of our results fails to disclose any frequent cause for a poor visual prognosis. Of possible causes for severe visual loss, keratoconus is relatively rare, and opacification at the apex of the cone due to breaks in Descemet membrane and hydrops (aqueous influx) is even more rare. Cataracts of visual significance are also rare, and are usually not present during early childhood when visual development takes place. Optic nerve hypoplasia occurs frequently but does not seem to cause serious visual loss in most cases. Retinal detachment can cause serious visual loss, but is quite rare. Nystagmus is not common and is usually relatively mild. Strabismus does not directly cause loss of visual acuity, although binocularity may be lost. However, strabismus is correctable either through refractive or surgical means. Similarly, ambylopia is completely reversible if treated appropriately and at an early age.

The most common and significant cause for visual loss associated with Down syndrome is refractive error. Since refractive errors can, with appropriate fixation conditions, be measured easily under cycloplegia, and since glasses are easily obtainable, there is little reason at present for refractive visual loss to be permitted to remain uncorrected in any but the most uncooperative and recalcitrant Down syndrome patient.

In conclusion, visual loss to a significant degree should be a rare, and usually an avoidable, event in Down syndrome. All children with Down syndrome should have early screening by an ophthalmologist well versed in dealing with disabled patients, and all indicated treatment should be promptly instituted to optimize visual outcome.

References

Ahmad, A., & Pruett, R.C. (1976). The fundus in Mongolism. *Archives of Ophthalmology, 94*, 772–776.

Awan, K.J. (1977). Uncommon ocular changes in Down syndrome (Mongolism). *Journal of Pediatric Ophthalmology, 14*, 215–216.

Brushfield, T. (1924). Mongolism. *British Journal of Diseases of Childhood, 21*, 241–258.

Cullen, J.F., & Butler, H.G. (1963). Mongolism and keratoconus. *British Journal of Ophthalmology, 47*, 321.

Donaldson, D.D. (1961). Significance of spotting of iris in mongoloids. *Archives of Ophthalmology, 65*, 26–31.

Down, J.L.H. (1866). Observations of ethnic classifications of idiots. *London Hospital Reports, 3*, 256.

Eissler, R., & Longenecker, L.P. (1962). The common eye findings in Mongolism. *American Journal of Ophthalmology, 54*, 398–406.

Engler, M. (1949). Mongolism. Bristol, England: J. Wright & Sons, Ltd.

Gannon, M.W., & Schimek, R.A. (1977). Down syndrome: A ten-year group study. *Annals of Ophthalmology*, 1493–1497.

Gifford, S.R. (1924). Congenital anomalies of lens as seen with slit lamp. *American Journal of Ophthalmology, 7*, 678–685.

Hiles, D.A., Hoyme, S.H., & McFarlane, F. (1974). Down syndrome and strabismus. *American Orthoptic Journal, 24*, 63–68.

Lambert, S.R., Hoyt, C.S., & Narakara, M.H. (1987). Optic nerve hypoplasia. *Survey of Ophthalmology, 32*, 1–9.

Last, R.J. (1968). *Wolff's anatomy of the eye and orbit (p. 146)*. London: H.K. Lewis & Co. Ltd.

Lejuene, J., Gauthier, M., & Turpin, R. (1959). *Les chromosomes humains en culture de tissues*, CR Acad Sc, *248*, 602–603.

Levinson, A., Friedeman, A., & Stamps, F. (1955). Variability of Mongolism. *Pediatrics*, *16*, 43–54.

Lowe, R.F. (1949). The eyes of Mongolism. *British Journal of Ophthalmology*, *33*, 131–154.

Lyle, W.M., Woodruff, M.E., & Zuccaro, V.S. (1972). A review of the literature on Down syndrome and an optometrical survey of 44 patients with the syndrome. *American Journal of Optometry Archives of the American Acadcmy of Optometry*, *49* (9), 715–727.

Oliver, C.A. (1891). A clinical study of the occular symptoms found in the so-called Mongolian type of idiocy. *Transactions of the American Ophthalmic Society*, *6*, Part I, 140–148.

Ormond, A.W. (1910). Notes on the ophthalmic conditions of forty-two Mongolian imbeciles. *Transactions of the Ophthalmic Society of the United Kingdom*, *32*, 69.

Peterson, R.A., & Walton, D.A. (1977). Optic nerve hypoplasia with good visual acuity and visual field defects: A study of children of diabetic mothers, *Archives of Ophthalmology*, *95*, 254–258.

Robb, R.M. (1977). Hemangioma of the eyelid associated with refractive error in childhood and infancy. *American Journal of Ophthalmology*, *83*, 52–58.

Schoen, M.J.A. (1828). *Handbuch der Pathologischen Anatomie des Menschlichen Auges*. Hamburg, Germany: Hoffman & Campe.

Shapiro, M.B., & France, T.D. (1985). The ocular features of Down syndrome. *American Journal of Ophthalmology*, *99*, 659–663.

Sheller, E., & Oster, J. (1951). Eye symptoms in Mongolism. *Acta Ophthalmologica*, *29*, 149–161.

Smith, J.L. (Ed.) (1980). Hypoplasia of the optic nerve and disk. *Neuro-ophthalmology Focus (p. 95)*. New York: Mason.

Solomons, G., Zellweger, H., Jahnke, P.G., Opitz, E. (1985). Four common eye signs in Mongolism. *American Journal of Diseases of Childhood*, *110*, 46–50.

Soberi, A., Sheridan, M., Leary, G.A., & Benjamin, B. (1960). Vision, visual acuity and ocular refraction of young men. *British Medical Journal*, *1*, 1394–1400.

Sutherland, G.A. (1899). *Practitioner*, 632.

Van der Scheer, W.M. (1927). Beitrage zur Kenntnis der Mongoloiden. *Missbildung, Klin Monatsbl f Augenheilk*, *62*, 155.

Von Ammon, F.A. quoted in Stewart, William B. (1984) Ophthalmic Plastic and Reconstructive surgery, San Francisco, California, American Academy of Ophthalmology, Publisher, 101 and Lowe, R.F. (see in reference section).

Wallis, R.E. (1951). Significance of Brushfield spots in diagnosis of Mongolism in infancy. *Archives of Disabilities of Children*, *26*, 495–500.

Walsh, F.B., & Hoyt, W.F. (1969). *Clinical neuro-ophthalmology (pp. 1, 70)*. Baltimore, Md.: Williams & Wilkins Co.

Williams, E.J. McCormick, A.Q., & Tischler, B. (1973). Retinal vessels in Down's syndrome. *Archives of Ophthalmology*, *89(4)*, 269–271.

Wolfflin, E. (1902). *Ein klinischer Beitrag zur kenntnis stinktur der Iris. Arch Augenheilk*, 45, 1–4.

4
Cardiac Conditions

L. Stephen Gordon

Introduction

Although the exact incidence of congenital heart disease (Spicer, 1984) in Down syndrome is not truly known, we can estimate that 40–50% of patients with this syndrome will have some form of congenital cardiac disease. The most common defect will be atrioventricular canal, either complete or partial, and the second most common defect will be ventricular septal defect. Ostium secundum atrial septal and tetralogy of Fallot are the other common cardiac defects, and the most common associated lesions are patent ductus arteriousus and pulmonary stenosis.

A study by Rowe and Uchida (1961) observed 70 patients with Down syndrome, of whom 36% had atrioventricular canal defects, 33% had ventricular septal defects, and 10% had patent ductus arteriousus, 9% had secundum artial septal defects, and 1% had tetralogy of Fallot. Of the 251 cases reported by Park et al. (1977), 45% had endocardial cushion defects, of which 27% had associated patent ductus arteriousus (PDA) and 17% had associated pulmonic stenosis; 31.9% had ventricular septal defects, of which 34% had associated patent ductus arteriosus and 22% had associated pulmonary stenosis. Of the 9.5% of patients with isolated atrial septal defects, 15% had associated patent ductus arteriosus. There were 6.4% of the patients who had tetralogy of Fallot. The review in 1973 by Tandon and Edwards of 55 cardiac specimens from subjects with Down syndrome, demonstrated that 47% had an associated PDA with their atrioventricular canal, and that 81% had an associated PDA with their ventricular septal defect. There were 60 percent of the patients who had a common atrioventricular canal, and 29% had an isolated ventricular septal defect. Tetralogy of Fallot occurred either alone or in association with a common atrioventricular canal 14.5% of the time.

The clinical recognition of congenital heart disease in infants with Down syndrome should be easy with the recent developments in two-dimensional echocardiography, Doppler flow analysis, and the recent introduction of color flow maps. Cardiac ultrasound may safely be performed before and/or after birth to identify patients with Down syndrome and congenital cardiac disease.

Survival associated with congenital cardiac malformation and Down syndrome may depend on early detection and diagnosis of this anomaly and the associated cardiac anomaly. The most common nonsurgical causes of death associated with Down syndrome and congenital cardiac malformation include congestive heart failure, hypoxic spells, Eisenmenger's syndrome, aspiration, or infective pneumonia. The overall significance of the problem is well defined by Greenwood and Nadas (1976), who reviewed the medical records from the Children's Hospital Medical Center in Boston from 1962 to 1973. Mortality was exceptionally high, 38% in all patients with endocardial cushion defect; and even higher, 52%, in those patients with complete atrioventricular canal. In patients with ventricular septal defect, mortality was 20%; it reached 42% in those patients with tetralogy of Fallot. The most common complication of congenital heart disease in this early series was pulmonary vascular obstructive disease. This appeared as early as 3 months of age in patients with complete atrioventricular canal, and as early as 11 months of age in patients with partial endocardial cushion defect. Only three patients with other left-to-right shunts, which included ventricular septal defect, ostium secundum artial septal defect, and isolated patent ductus arteriosus, did not have significant pulmonary artery hypertension. Pulmonary vascular obstructive disease was present in 11 of 13 patients with pulmonary artery hypertension. All of the patients with cyanosis and tetralogy of Fallot had severe systemic desaturation. Surgical success was quite limited and medical management was clearly unsuccessful. Pulmonary artery banding for complete endocardial cushion defect was in general unsuccessful, as one might expect in an obligatory shunt. In general, medical management of all lesions with significant shunts was unsuccessful, and surgical management at an earlier age might have prevented significant cardiac complications.

A high Prenatal index of suspicion may help. The review of Greenwood and Nadas, from the regional infant cardiac program of New England, 1968 to 1973, demonstrated that of all infants critically ill with heart disease, 4% may be expected to have Down syndrome. This extrauterine incidence of congenital heart disease as a marker for Down syndrome compares unfavorably with the intrauterine diagnosis of this syndrome in association with congenital heart disease. For example, the expected incidence of Down syndrome in those fetuses with congenital heart disease is significantly higher than 4%, indicating that there is significant fetal wastage before birth.

Moreover, the high incidence of other associated problems such as recurrent respiratory infections and congenital abnormalities often affects the clinical outcome of children with Down syndrome and congenital cardiac disease. Comprehensive medical programs that pay attention to all organ systems may limit the effect of these problems on the long-term clinical outcome.

Therefore, recent advances in neonatal and prenatal diagnosis and therapy, which include open cardiac surgical repair at a younger age, have led to the survival of more infants with Down syndrome. As these children grow up, however, adolescents and young adults will obviously be seen with a spectrum of cardiac defects that may range from minor adult problems such as mitral valve prolapse and minor cardiac arrhythmias to the more severe unoperated patients with polycythemia, Eisenmenger's syndrome, and severe pulmonary vascular obstructive disease.

Patient Population

In our study of cardiac conditions in persons with Down syndrome, the patient population is that described in the introduction and Appendix 1. The vast majority of these patients had cardiac care provided in another clinical setting. Cardiology consultation was available, either by case finding, parental request, or referral. Diagnostic categories were established by both parental information and review of prior medical records, including surgical operative notes. The study was retrospective. The patient population can be defined as alive and well, and therefore exclusive of all new cases of serious congenital cardiac malformation admitted to the hospital for intercurrent illness or diagnosis.

Methods

All parents were provided a questionnaire with the following questions:

- Was there history of a heart murmur?
- Was there history of cyanosis?
- Was there history of fainting?
- Was there history of shortness of breath with exertion?
- Was there history of chest pain?
- Was there history of palpitations?
- Was there history of prior heart surgery?
- Was there history of cardiac catheterization?

All patients were evaluated by a pediatrician, who also evaluated the information provided on the cardiac data questionnaires. Based on this clinical evaluation, patients were then referred for cardiac consultation if deemed necessary. The clinical cardiologist did not see all patients with congenital heart disease, and data as to the physical performance and cardiac status were available only on those patients seen.

Results

A total of 77 out of 190 patients were designated as potentially having congenital cardiac disease (Table 4.1). Fourteen patients had a functional cardiac murmur and were excluded from the disease category. This left 63 patients with a congenital cardiac abnormality. There were 28 males and 35 females with congenital heart disease. Twelve patients were less than 1 year of

TABLE 4.1. Heart disease in Down syndrome (N = 190).

Problem	N	%
Functional heart murmur	14	8
Congenital heart disease	63	38
AV canal (complete/partial)	21	
Ventricular septal defect	20	
Atrial septal defect, Ostium secundum	6	
Mitral value prolapse	3	
Complete heart block	1	
Tetralogy of fallot	1	
Irregular rhythm	1	
Aortic valve stenosis	1	
Mitral atresia	1	
Patent ductus arteriosus	8	

age, 33 patients were between 1 and 5 years of age, 10 patients were between 5 and 10 years of age, and 9 patients were older than 10 years of age. Twenty-one patients had atriovenricular canal defects, either complete or partial, 20 patients had isolated ventricular septal defects, 6 patients had ostium secundum atrial septal defects, 3 patients had mitral valve prolapse and one of these patients also had complete heart block, one patient had tetralogy of Fallot, one patient had an irregular cardiac rhythm, one patient had aortic valve stenosis, one patient had mitral valve atresia with ventricular septal defect and coarctation, and one patient had pulmonary valve stenosis. There were 8 patients who had a patent ductus arteriousus and only 2 of these occurred as an isolated lesion. Five occurred in association with an atrioventricular canal defect, and one occurred in association with an ostium secundum atrial septal defect.

Discussion of Diagnosis and Management of Common Cardiac Lesions

The endocardial cushions first appear in the 6 mm embryo as young mesenchymal outpouchings. They are superior to the conoventricular fold, and they begin to close the opening between the superior primitive artiae and the primitive ventricles (Van Mierop, 1976). By approximately 9–10 mm embryo size, the cushions have rapidly increased so that they meet and fuse, and smaller masses of endocardial cushion type tissue will appear on the right and left lateral borders of the atrioventricular canal and will eventually form the true atrioventricular canals. By 17 mm in length, the cardiac septation process is complete except for the final closure of the atrial septum. The complete form of endocardial cushion defect or common atrioventricular canal is the result of nonunion of the endocardial cushions. The final anatomy is an ostium primum defect low in the atrial septum and a large ventricular septal defect communicating with the ostium primum defect. There is no division of the atrioventricular ring into a separate mitral or tricuspid valve orifice, and there is, therefore, a single atrioventricular valve divided into anterior and posterior leaflets. One can visualize the defect as a large central hole within the cardiac skeleton that allows for complete mixing of all four chambers. Three types of the complete form of atrioventricular canal were defined by Rastelli, Kirklin, and Titus (1966). In type I, the anterior leaflet is divided and attached to the ventricular septum. In type II, the anterior leaflet is divided but not attached to the ventricular septum; the membranous ventricular septum is also involved and the ventricular septal component is usually large. In type III, the anterior leaflet is not divided, nor is it attached to the ventricular septum. The membranous septum is again absent.

Clinical Evaluation

The initial high pulmonary artery pressure in the newborn infant may interfere with any significant left-to-right shunt and the infant may be asymptomatic. The initial clinical findings usually associated with a large left-to-right shunt in the newborn infant, such as a bounding precordium or cardiac murmur, are generally absent. By 4 to 8 weeks of life, pulmonary arterial pressure begins to fall and the left-to-right shunt ensues. At this time, the first cardiac sound is accentuated at the left lower sternal border. The pulmonary component of the second heart sound is loud and at times fuses with the aortic component of the second heart sound. A systolic ejection murmur along the left sternal border indicates the increase in pulmonary blood flow, and an apical pansystolic murmur radiating to the axilla hallmarks mitral valve regurgitation. A pulmonary-to-systemic blood flow ratio usually greater than 2:1 follows, and there is a middiastolic rumble over the left lower sternal border or cardiac apex. Most infants are tachypneic with hepatomegaly and may be mildly cyanotic due to the complete intracardiac mixing of blood and a "washing machine" effect.

The electrocardiogram (Figure 4.1) shows a left superior axis, usually less than—90 degrees, and one may find combined atrial hypertrophy. There is usually prolongation of the PR interval and combined ventricular hypertrophy, although left or right ventricular hypertrophy may predominate. The chest film demonstrates moderate to severe cardiomegaly, with enlargement of the cardiac silhousette, particularly to the left, and at times dilation of the main pulmonary artery segment. There is a significant increase in pulmonary arterial vascular markings. Two-dimensional echocardiography, particularly with Doppler flow and color flow mapping, defines the anatomy. The deficiency of the atrial and ventricular septae are best visualized in the apical and precordial four-chambered views, and the anatomy of the atrioventricular valves is evident. Attachments or nonattachments of the anterior leaflet (Figure 4.2) to the ventricular septi are clearly visualized in the apical four-

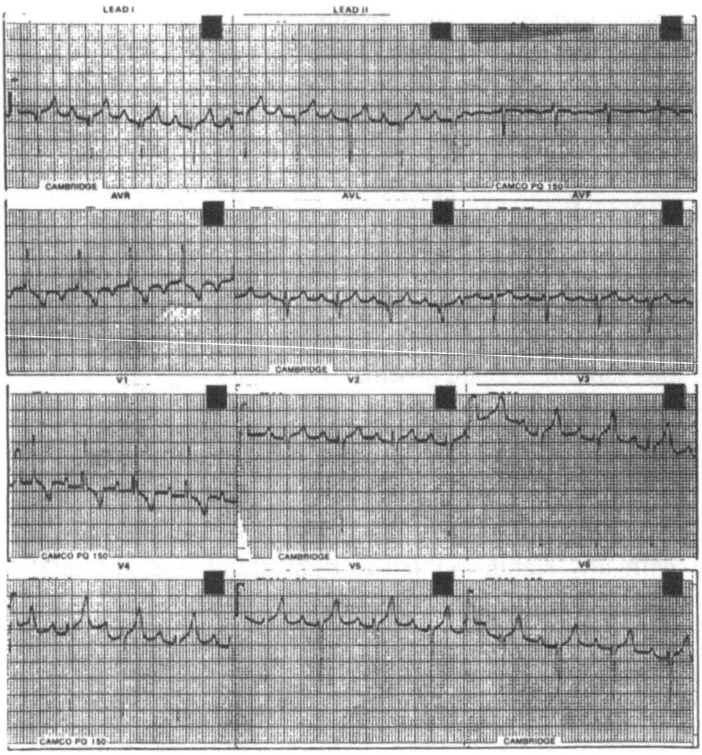

FIGURE 4.1. Electrocardiogram demonstrating the usual findings in a complete atrioventricular canal defect. There is prolongation of the PR interval, a left superior axis counter clockwise frontal phone loop, (Q waves in leads I and AVL), an incomplete right bundle branch block pattern and right ventricular hypertrophy. The patient had associated Eisenmenger's syndrome.

chambered view. Doppler interrogation (Figure 4.3) of the atrioventricular valves demonstrate the presence and severity of mitral valve regurgitation and/or tricuspid valve regurgitation in association with a large left-to-right atrial-ventricular shunt. The apical four-chamber view of the echocardiogram also clearly defines whether one or the other ventricle is dominant and helps in the decisions for surgical management. Color flow mapping may be helpful in the definition of an associated patent ductus arteriosus, however, it is suggested that descending aortography be used to clearly define whether or not a ductus arteriosus is present. The patients at greatest risk for progression of pulmonary artery hypertension to pulmonary vascular obstructive disease are those patients with a patent ductus arteriosus in association with the atrioventricular canal defect. Complete right and left cardiac catheterization help in the delineation of the physiology and determination of the pulmonary arterial vascular resistance. Angiography, particularly of the left ventricle in

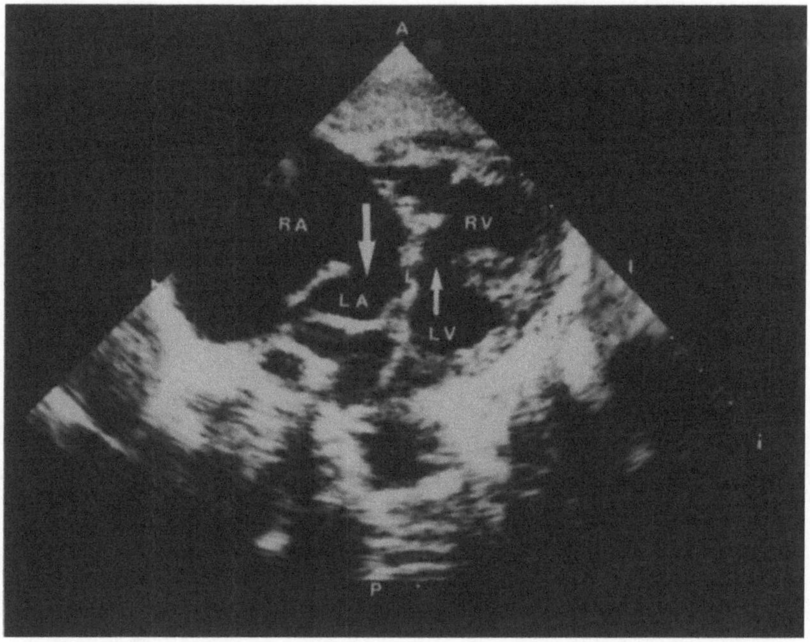

FIGURE 4.2. A two-dimensional echocardiogram demonstrating a complete atrioventricular canal defect of the type III variety. There is no attachment of the common anterior leaflet to the ventricular septum, and the ostium primum atrial septal defect and endocardial cushion type ventricular septal defect are quite large. There is massive right and left atrial dilatation due to the severe AV valve regurgitation.
Abbreviations: A = anterior; P = posterior; I = inferior; RA = right atrium; LA = left atrium; RV = Right ventricle; LV = left ventricle; Large arrow = atrial component of defect; Small arrow = ventricular component of defect; and L = the common leaflet lies between the arrows.

the left anterior oblique cranial angulated view, defines the position and size of the ventricular septal defect, rules out muscular defects, and angulation of the X-ray beam into an apical four-chamber view defines the anatomy of the atrial septal defect. The combination of cardiac catheterization and careful two-dimensional echocardiography are necessary to time the surgical repair, and are also helpful in formulating the long-term prognosis and plan.

Patients with cardiac failure usually respond to Digoxin®, Lasix®, and Aldactone®. If AV valve regurgitation is significant, afterload reduction with Captopril®, will help in reducing the degree of AV valve insufficiency. The correction of anemia and infection is critical in the management of these patients.

The partial or transitional form of endocardial cushion defect is also known as an incomplete atrioventricular canal defect. A large, ostium primum-type

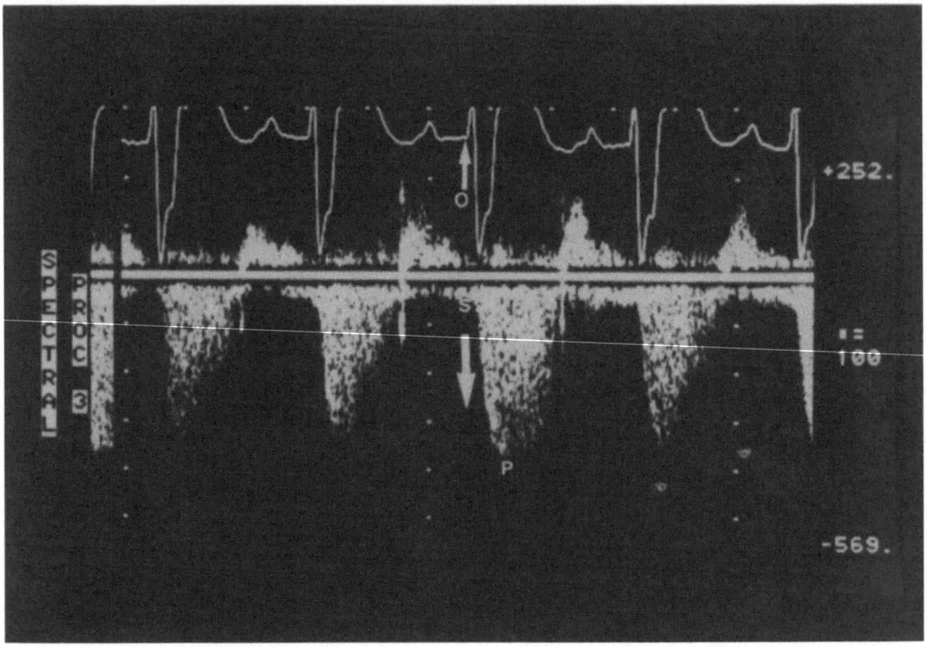

FIGURE 4.3. A continuous wave Doppler flow tracing demonstrating a high-velocity pansystolic regurgitant flow profile in a patient with an atrioventricular canal defect. The regurgitant fraction begins at the onset of ventricular systole (0) and ends at the end of ventricular systole. P = peak regurgitant velocity across the left sided atrioventricular valve; S marks the beginning of systolic regurgitant jet; Arrow = direction of pansystolic regurgitant flow. An EKG lead II is displayed above.

atrial septal defect is usually at the crux of the heart and some deformity, a cleft, is usually present in both right and left atrioventricular valves. The size of the ventricular septal defect is smaller due to a greater deficiency of the atrial, rather than the ventricular septum and the mitral and tricuspid valves may be only mildly incompetent. These children will present with a similar course as described, but somewhat less cardiac failure at 4 to 8 weeks of age. Cyanosis is less frequent; however, cardiac examination may be similar to that for the complete form of endocardial cushion defect.

The electrocardiogram will show the same leftward and superior axis with a counterclockwise frontal plane loop and combined ventricular hypertrophy. The chest film usually shows moderate to severe cardiomegaly and increased pulmonary blood flow. Two-dimensional echocardiography best defines the anatomy, and cardiac catheterization best defines the physiology. Again, it is suggested that once cardiac failure has been diagnosed in these patients, careful attempts be made to rule out a patent ductus arteriosus.

It is important to mention the role of the ductus arteriosus in patients with a large left-to-right shunt and AV valve regurgitation. An obligatory intracardiac shunt is not dependent on the resistance or impedance downstream, which is defined by the pulmonary arterial vascular resistance. For example, with the ductus arteriosus open, aortic pressure is communicated to the pulmonary arterial vascular bed raising pulmonary arterial pressure, and concomitant with that increase in pressure there is a left-to-right ductal shunt. There will be volume overload of the ventricles which is independent of pulmonary artery pressure however, due to the large interatrial communication. Also the incompetent AV valve serves as a "pop off" for ventricular ejection (the low-pressure artial sink), since the pulmonary resistance downstream of the right ventricle will be higher than either atrial pressure.

This physiologic consequence of disturbed anatomy results in the worst possible situation: pulmonary arterial hypertension from the PDA and VSD concomitant with a volume overloaded heart from the ASD and AV valve regurgitation. The net result is poor systemic perfusion, low systemic cardiac output, and massively increased pulmonary blood flow. Even under the best of circumstances, that is, full digitalization and diuretic therapy with afterload reduction, the ventricles are working at maximum efficiency, and any stress that requires an increase in cardiac output, such as fever, DPT injection, diarrhea, vomiting, or a flu-like syndrome, may result in a significant drop in cardiac output due to an already compromised circulatory state. For this reason we suggest that once the ductus arteriosus is identified, it be surgically ligated or closed with an intravascular occluder device, since this will improve medical management, and may allow corrective surgery to be deferred, often until the child is 6 months of age.

The most incomplete form of atrioventricular canal defect is the ostium primum atrial septal defect. This low atrial septal defect is situated at the crux of the heart in contact with both the tricuspid and mitral valve (there is usually a tiny defect in the ventricular septum as well, but this is inconsequential). This defect is present in only a few patients with Down syndrome and may not be present until 3 to 4 years of age, when cardiac output may increase and a significant pulmonary flow murmur is heard. There may or may not be anatomic evidence for a cleft in the formation of the mitral valve so that mitral valve regurgitation may indeed be associated.

On physical examination, the patients often have a hyperactive precordium with a palpable right ventricular impulse. There is a grade II/VI to III/VI systolic ejection murmur best heard at the left midsternal border with radiation toward the pulmonary outflow tract. The cardiac second sound is usually a fixed split with little or no variation noted, and the pulmonary components of the second heard sound is soft. There is usually a grade II/VI diastolic flow rumble best heard over the xiphoid process; this rumble is accentuated by placing the patient in the supine position and increasing the venous return. An apical to axillary pansystolic murmur suggests the presence of AV valve regurgitation, particularly through a cleft in the mitral valve. The electrocardiograph usually demonstrates prolongation of the PR interval, right ventricular hypertrophy, and a leftward and superior frontal plane axis with a counterclockwise frontal plane loop. The chest film usually defines mild cardiomegaly with prominence of the main pulmonary artery segment and increased pulmonary blood flow.

Two-dimensional echocardiography is usually adequate to define the anatomy and physiology, although careful Doppler flow analysis must be performed to rule out a left-to-right ductal shunt. The degree of AV valve regurgitation can easily be defined by Doppler or color flow analysis, and a large atrial septal defect will be defined in the ostium primum position. The cleft in the mitral valve can often be seen and sometimes there is associated anterior, inferior displacement of the mitral valve that one similarly sees in the more severe form of atrioventricular canal defect.

Management is relatively easy since these patients often have no symptoms, and elective surgical repair is usually successful. Those patients with significant AV valve regurgitation may require digoxin and diuretics.

In our series, ventricular septal defect was the second most common lesion associated with Down syndrome. The classical course of a ventricular septal defect is well known. Usually, the infant with a large ventricular septal defect has no symptoms due to the high pulmonary arterial pressures present in the neonatal period. As the pulmonary arterial vascular resistance begins to fall, a large left-to-right shunt ensues and the infant may present with poor feeding, diaphoresis, cyanosis, ashen gray color, respiratory distress, anemia, and/or pneumonia. Cardiac examination will demonstrate a loud pansystolic murmur associated with a loud first heart sound and a narrowly split second heart sound. There is often an apical diastolic flow rumble. There may be bilateral rales due to left heart failure and significant hepatomegaly.

The electrocardiogram will demonstrate a normal frontal plane axis (0 to 180 degrees). Combined ventricular hypertrophy is common. The chest film will demonstrate moderate to severe cardiomegaly and increased pulmonary vascular markings. Two-dimensional echocardiography again clearly defines the status of the endocardial cushions and the AV valve so that this most common cardiac lesion can be ruled out and ventricular septal defect can be defined. One must again search carefully for an associated patent ductus arteriosus or, in some cases, associated pulmonary outflow obstruction and a developing course similar to tetralogy of Fallot.

Cardiac catheterization is often necessary to define the true anatomy and pulmonary arterial vascular resistance so that one may establish a long-range plan. Again, a left ventriculogram in the cranial angulated left anterior oblique view is the best procedure to define the size and location of the ventricular septal defect. A descending aortogram will be necessary to rule out a left-to-right ductal shunt.

Tetralogy of Fallot is the most common cyanotic cardiac defect associated with Down syndrome. Infants with this defect often present in the newborn period with mild to moderate cyanosis and tachypnea. This defect consists of pulmonary outflow tract stenosis, usually at the pulmonary annulus, pulmonary valve, and particularly at the infundibular region, a large infundibular ventricular septal defect so positioned that there is no superior rim and there is significant aortic valve overriding due to the leftward and anterior positioning of the crista supraventricularis. The tetralogy is completed by right ventricular hypertrophy, which is secondary to the pulmonary outflow tract obstruction. The net result is that the right ventricular (desaturated) blood is ejected through the ventricular septal defect directly into the ascending aorta, and cyanosis ensues. All patients with tetralogy of Fallot have similar but not identical symptoms; therefore, clinical management will depend on individual case analysis. Many patients have minimal cyanosis and may be managed with careful follow-up until they are at an appropriate size and age for repair. We tend to choose 18 months for the previously asymptomatic child. Surgical repair may be preceded by surgical palliation, which in most circumstances, includes a modified Blalock-Taussing shunt provided by a 5 or 6 mm Gortex graft anastomosed from either subclavian artery to the ipsilateral pulmonary artery. The "shunt" provides adequate pulmonary blood flow distal to the pulmonary outflow obstruction and allows both the child and the pulmonary arteries to grow appropriately. The ideal "shunted" patient would not require complete repair until between the age of 18 and 36 months. In the Boston series, 8.3% of the Down syndrome patients had tetralogy of Fallot; in the Park series, 6.4%.

Pulmonary Arterial Vascular Disease

We have already alluded to the relationship of the ductus arteriosus and pulmonary arterial vascular disease in association with other significant cardiac lesions in Down syndrome. It is generally accepted that pulmonary arterial hypertension, and thus the future development of pulmonary vascular obstructive disease, occurs earlier in infants with Down syndrome than in normal infants with similar cardiac defects. Although the actual etiology remains unclear, Levine and Simpser (1982) report the effects of alveolar hypoventilation and corpulmonale associated with chronic airway obstruction in infants with Down syndrome. Loughlin, Wyme and Victoria (1981) reported sleep apnea as a possible cause of pulmonary hypertension in Down syndrome. Conney and Thurlbeck (1982) used morphometric analysis to demonstrate pulmonary hypoplasia in Down syndrome. They demonstrated a diminished number of alveoli and enlarged alveoli and alveolar ducts, associated with a small alveolar surface area. There appears to be inadequate alveolarization of the terminal lung units distal to the respiratory bronchioles. This reduced internal surface of the lungs in patients with Down syndrome will lead to alveolar hypoventilation, hypoxemia, hypercarbia, and acidemia.

These metabolic abnormalities can produce pulmonary artery hypertension. Yamaki, Horiuschi, and Sekino (1983) demonstrated that pulmonary arterial parenchymal changes developed early in patients with Down syndrome and congenital heart disease, and the media of small pulmonary arteries in simple cardiac anomalies with Down syndrome was thinner than the media in cases without this syndrome. The authors conclude that "retarded development of medial hypertrophy in Down syndrome, in response to pulmonary artery hypertension, appears to make the pulmonary arteries susceptible to even a moderate pressure load and appears to be responsible for early development of severe parenchymal changes."

In addition to the anatomic alveolar, pulmonary arterial abnormalities, children with Down syndrome are more susceptible to pulmonary infections. Gastroesophageal reflux with aspiration has been implicated in some patients, as has the Down syndrome child's inability to resist some pulmonary infections (Weesner & Rosenthal, 1983).

It has been well known for a long time that chronic upper airway obstruction can lead to pulmonary hypertension, particularly in Down syndrome. Levine and Simpser (1982) have reported four infants with Down syndrome, cor pulmonale, and heart failure who have benefitted only by tracheostomy. These patients demonstrated chronic tonsillar and adenoidal hypertrophy and symptoms similar to sleep apnea. Levine and Simpser (1982) concluded that infants with Down syndrome may be predisposed to upper airway obstruction by virtue of hypoplasia of facial and oropharyngeal structures and generalized hypotonia. Additional obstructive elements may be contributed by hypertrophied lymphoid tissue, excessive secretions, and glossoptosis.

The cumulative effect of upper airway obstruction, recurrent bronchospasm and infections, pulmonary hypoplasia, and underdeveloped pulmonary arterioles, a left-to-right cardiac shunt, and chronic cardiac failure will be pulmonary arterial hypertension, and with it, early and accelerated pulmonary arterial vascular disease.

The clinical diagnosis of pulmonary arterial vascular disease in the young patient, particularly a child less than a year of age, may be difficult. A loud pulmonic closure may appear late in the development of pulmonary artery hypertension, and the electrocardiogram may already demonstrate right ventricular hypertrophy. Pulmonary oligemia, on chest film, also may appear late in the development of pulmonary artery hypertension. Echocardiographic features of pulmonary arterial hypertension and/or pulmonary arterial vascular disease are not yet accurate enough to predict reversibility or irreversibility of the hypertension.

Careful cardiac catheterization with evaluation of pulmonary arterial response to both oxygen and priscoline remains the hallmark of diagnosis for pulmonary artery hypertension. It is important to note that there are some patients with Down syndrome who have irreversible pulmonary arterial vascular disease before 1 year of age.

Clinical Management of the Infant with Down Syndrome and Cardiac Disease

The initial problem for any congenital cardiac lesion is diagnosis. It is presently recommended that all patients who have proven trisomy 21 by amniocentesis have fetal echocardiography, and all fetuses who have atrioventricular canal by cardiac ultrasound have amniocentesis. Prenatal diagnosis of cardiac disease, particularly atrioventricular canal, will assist in the immediate neonatal management and care of those infants. It is imperative, however, that all newborns with Down syndrome have sufficient diagnostic evaluation to exclude congenital heart disease. Cardiac ultrasound testing in the neonatal period will reveal a 40–50% rate of cardiac problems when all babies with Down syndrome are studied. It is fallacious to assume that asymptomatic infants with Down syndrome have no congenital cardiac disease.

Once the diagnosis has been established, clinical management includes digoxin, diuretics, and afterload reduction. We have already discussed the need to manage anemia, respiratory insufficiency, and chronic and recurrent infections. Gastroesophageal reflux and sleep apena may be problematic. Once the patient with Down syndrome develops congestive cardiac failure, then it becomes necessary to rule out an associated patent ductus arteriosus and to define carefully the intracardiac anatomy and physiology. Cardiac catheterization in the patients with congestive cardiac failure should be performed before 6 months of age, and descending aortography must be performed to rule out a patent ductus arteriosus. If necessary, one may administer priscoline and oxygen as pulmonary vasodilators in the catheterization laboratory to assess the pulmonary vasculature.

Surgical techniques (Figure 4.4) have improved to the point that, if necessary, cardiopulmonary bypass with deep hypothermia and cardioplegia will permit complete intracardiac repair at essentially any age. In 37 patients with Down syndrome at Children's Hospital of Los Angeles, operated on between 1980 and 1986 for atrioventricular canal or ventricular septal defect, the mortality rate was 13.5% (Wells & Lindesmith, 1987, Personal communication). However, a significant number of immediate postoperative complications occurred, which included pulmonary atelectasis and infiltrates, persistent pulmonary hypertension, postoperative pneumonia, bradycardia, and cardiac arrest, severe bleeding, bilateral pleural effusion, and residual defects. Long-term follow-up demonstrated that residual mitral valve regurgitation was the most common recurrent problem. Berger et al., (1978) have demonstrated by actuarial analysis that only 54% of infants with unoperated atrioventricular canal will survive to 6 months of age, 35% to 12 months of age, 15% to 24 months of age, and 4% to 5 years of age. In their institute, surgical mortality was 17% by 12 months of age. It appears clear that life expectancy without surgery for this cardiac defect is grim, and that early surgical intervention is the best alternative.

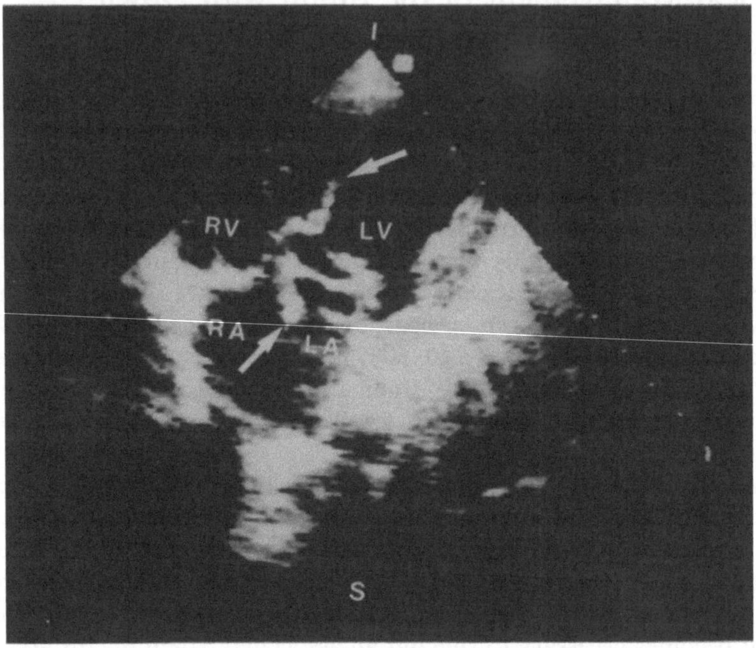

FIGURE 4.4. An apical four-chambered view of a two-dimensional echocardiogram demonstrating a repaired atrioventricular canal defect. The repaired atrioventricular valves are closed. The arrows point to the large atrioventricular septal patch, which connects the inferior margin of the atrial septum to the superior crest of the ventricular septum.
I = inferior; S = superior; RA = right atrium; RV = right ventricle; LA = left atrium; LV = left ventricle.

Ethical Issues in the Management of Infants with Down Syndrome and Congenital Heart Disease

J.C. Murdoch (1985) reviewed the statement published in the *British Medical Journal* in 1981: "If the child is one of the one-quarter of newborns with Down syndrome with congenital defects of the heart or other organs, then treatment may reasonably be withheld." He compared 84 children with Down syndrome and no congenital heart disease to 48 children with both diagnoses. The parameters included total contacts with physicians and new contacts for respiratory problems. There was essentially no specific difference in the two groups when corrected for one or two patients who had multiple visits. Although the study included only survivors of the neonatal period, there were 10 patients (7%) of the group who had complex cardiac malformations. He concluded:

> A comparison of children with Down syndrome classified according to having congenital heart disease has shown no differences in contact with the general practitioner, new episodes of respiratory illness, acute admission to hospital, or mortality over the period studied. It is suggested that the prognostic significance of coincidental congenital heart disease in Down syndrome be questioned.

No doubt Dr. Murdoch has presented important information. However, management of the infant with Down syndrome and severe congenital heart disease does present a different problem. According to Kirklin and Barratt Boyes (1986), the chance of surviving with an atrioventricular canal to 6 months of age is only 50% untreated. The issue, therefore, is what to do in the first 6 months of age, not later. Sondheimer, Bjrum, and Blackman (1985) looked at two groups of patients with atrioventricular canal. They reviewed referral patterns for patients with atrioventricular canal and Down syndrome or atrioventricular canal and no Down syndrome. Of the 8 children without Down syndrome, all were referred before one year of age, and of the 28 Down syndrome children, 10 were referred after one year of age. Surgical intervention was not possible in 5 of those 10 patients. They conclude:

> ...since complete atrioventricular canal is known to progress to pulmonary vascular obstructive disease at an early age, it is not surprising that half of those patients referred after 1 year of age had become inoperable because of this complication. We therefore concluded that in spite of the severity of complete atrioventricular canal, some children with Down syndrome and this heart condition are being denied standard cardiac care by the process of late referral.

It should be clear that neglect of the patient with Down syndrome and cardiac disease is not prudent. Patients who survive with complete atrioventricular canal and pulmonary vascular obstructive disease are significantly worse off than their surviving peers who have received treatment. One only has to follow, longitudinally, children with Down syndrome and atrioventricular canal and pulmonary vascular disease into their early 20s to realize the devastating nature of this illness. These children often must use a wheelchair, are persistently short of breath, cyanotic, and polycythemic. They may develop right heart failure. Clinical manifestations of their chronic hypoxemia include visual disturbances, severe headaches, dyspnea on any exertion, chest pain, syncope, cardiac dysrhythmias, and in some cases, associated bleeding tendency. There is no doubt that the quality of life in the unoperated patient who develops pulmonary vascular obstructive disease is poor.

Summary

This study reviews the spectrum of cardiovascular disease associated with Down syndrome. For a complete review of cardiology textbooks on cardiovascular disease in children, and on cardiovascular surgery, see Kirklin and Barratt-Boyes (1986), Perloff (1987), and Adams and Emmanouilides (1983).

We suggest that all infants with Down syndrome have a two-dimensional echocardiogram after birth (if they have not had one before birth) to completely define their cardiac anatomy, since these patients may be asymptomatic for 4 to 8 weeks. Overall, this test should reveal cardiac defects in 40–50% of all infants with Down syndrome. Medical management of Down syndrome and significant cardiovascular disease is usually possible for 6 months to 1 year, when surgical management becomes necessary. Of particular importance in children with Down syndrome is the management of noncardiac problems, to avoid the attendant cardiac stress and need for increased cardiac output. Antimicrobial prophylaxis for dental or surgical procedures should be instituted for all cardiac patients with Down syndrome. Older children with polycythemia and cardiovascular disease may require intermittent oxygen, periodic red cell volume reduction, and treatment for cardiac failure. Equal care should be provided for all patients, whether they have Down syndrome or not, since a lack of intervention may result in either mortality or a severely compromised quality of life if the child survives.

References

Adams, F.H., & Emmanouilides, G.C. (1983). *Heart disease in infants, children, and adolescents*, Baltimore, Md.: Williams and Wilkins.

Berger, T.J., Blackstone, E.H., Kirklin, J.W., Bargeron, L.M., Hazelring, J.B., & Turner, M.E. (1978). Survival and probability of cure without and with operation in complete atrioventricular canal. *Annual of Thorasic Surgery, 27*, 104–111.

Conney, T.P., & Thurlbeck, W.M. (1982) Pulmonary hypoplasia in Down syndrome. *New England Journal of Medicine, 307*, 1170–1173.

Greenwood, R.D., & Nadas, A.S. (1976). The clinical course of cardiac disease in Down syndrome. *Pediatrics, 58*, 893–897.

Kirklin, J.W., & Barratt-Boyes, B.G. (1986). *Cardiac Surgery*. New York: John Wiley & Sons.

Levine, O.R., & Simpser, M. (1982). Alveolar hypoventilation in cor pulmonale associated with chronic airway obstruction in infants with Down syndrome. *Clinical Pediatrics, 21*, 25–29.

Loughlin, G.N., Wynne, J.W., & Victorica, B.E. (1981). Sleep apnea as a possible cause of pulmonary hypertension of Down syndrome. *Journal of Pediatrics, 98*, 435–437.

Murdoch, J.C. (1985). Congenital heart disease as a significant factor in the morbidity of children with Down syndrome. *Journal of Mental Deficiency Research, 29*, 147–151.

Park, S.C., Matthews, R.A., Zuberbuhler, B. Jr., Rowe, R.D., Neches, W.H., & Lenox, C.C. (1977). Down syndrome with congenital heart malformation. *American Journal of Diseases of Children, 131*, 29–33.

Perloff, J.K. (1987). *The clinical recognition of congenital heart disease*. Philadelphia: W.B. Saunders.

Rastelli, G.C., Kirklin, J.W., & Titus, J.L. (1966). Anatomic observations on complete form of persistent common atrioventricular canal with special reference to atrioventricular valves. *Mayo Clinic Proceedings, 41*, 296–308.

Rowe, R.D., & Uchida, I.A. (1961). Cardiac malformation in Mongolism. *American Journal of Medicine, 31*, 726–735.

Sondheimer, H.M., Byrum, C.J., & Blackman, M.S. (1985). Unequal cardiac care for children with Down syndrome. *American Journal of Diseases of Children, 139*, 68–70.

Spicer, R.L. (1984). Cardiovascular disease in Down syndrome. *The Pediatric Clinics of North America, 31* (6), 1331–1343.

Tandon, R., & Edwards, J. (1973). Cardiac malformations associated with Down Syndrome. *Circulation, 47*, 1349–1355.

Van Mierop, L.H.S. (1976). *Embryology of the atrioventricular canal region and pathogenesis of endocardial cushion defects in atrioventricular canal defects (pp. 1–2).* R.H. Feldt (Ed.), Philadelphia: W.B. Saunders.

Weesner, K.M., & Rosenthal, A. (1983). Gastroesophageal reflux in association with congenital heart disease. *Clinical Pediatrics, 22*, 424–426.

Yamaki, S. Horiuschi, T., & Sekino, Y. (1983). Quantitative analysis of pulmonary vascular disease in simple cardiac anomalies with Down syndrome. *American Journal of Cardiology, 51*, 1502–1506.

5
Dental Problems

Oariona Lowe

Introduction

Individuals with Down syndrome have a number of developmental problems that raise barriers to routine delivery of dental care. Sources of dental treatment for these individuals has in the past been generally limited to medical institutions and dental schools. In the past, many dentists in private practice lacked adequate understanding and skills in the management of these patients, and were hesitant to offer dental treatment. Today, however, more and more private dental practitioners are willing to treat the individual with Down syndrome, due to improved operating efficiency, the use of auxilliaries, new dental materials, and improved patient management techniques.

Dental Evaluation of the Individual Down Syndrome

When seeing the child with Down syndrome for the first time, the dentist should take a complete and updated medical history, including information on current medications that the patient is taking. The dentist should seek information from the physician as to the existence of significant medical problems, a history of past surgery, and a history of past allergies. In addition, he or she needs to know whether there is any neuromotor involvement, history of seizures, drug therapy, visual or auditory defects, an estimate of intelligence level, and most important, whether the child has a history of congenital heart disease. A large percentage (40%) of children with this syndrome present with some form of congenital heart problems. These patients must be placed on antibiotic prophylaxis before any treatment is started (Greenwood & Nadus, 1976). The standard regimen is Penicillin V, 1 gram by mouth one hour before procedure, then 500 mg six hours after the initial dose, doubling the doses for the patient greater than 27 kg. There are special regimens for individuals not able to take oral medication, requiring maximal protection such as prothetic value, and those allergic to penicillin. If there is a history of blood dyscrasias, dental treatment may need to be limited to procedures that cause minimal bleeding in which local hemorrhage can be controlled.

Information taken as part of the dental history should include the date of the last dental examination, history of dental infection and gum disease, how often the teeth are brushed, and whether the patient can brush his or her own teeth. Classifying the patient's disability according to type and being aware of her/his physical impairments are important. Since the patient's level of cognitive functioning is often significantly affected, it is recommended that the patient be approached at his or her cognitive level, rather than on the basis of chronological age. If time is spent during the initial appointment to allow the child to become acquainted with the dentist and dental staff, fewer behavior problems will occur during future visits.

It is important to note that the dentist should take the time to explain procedures to the patient in a manner that he or she can understand. There is no "proper" approach or technique in delivering dental care to the patient with Down syndrome. The dentist's approach to the patient should be friendly, sympathetic, firm, and always completely confident. The child can sense a lack of assurance and this feeling can initiate an adverse attitude. For this reason, the dentist should display patience and persistence, a friendly relationship, and an atmosphere of confidence with procedures and examination. The aim of successful treatment is a team effort between the dentist, dental staff, and the child. To further this aim, the patient should be encouraged to ask questions and all procedures should be demonstrated at a level appropriate to the cognitive level of the individual.

The behavior of the child in the dental chair will ultimately determine the best approach. Sedation with an agent such as chloral hydrate is an option, but behavior management is always the first approach. If sedation is necessary, behavior techniques are always required in conjunction with such sedation. If sedation is unsuccessful, some individuals will need hospitalization (day surgery) with general anesthesia for dental care. However, after gathering the necessary information by means of a thorough history and a straightforward attempt at establishing rapport with the child, most children with Down syndrome can be treated effectively and efficiently within the normal routine of the dental office.

Patient Population

In this study of persons with Down syndrome, 188 individuals ranging from infancy to 19 years of age were evaluated by a pedodontist. There were slightly more females than males (98 females; 90 males). It was assumed that individuals younger than 2 years of age (70 individuals) had no or minimal teeth, and that dental findings were essentially normal. The remaining 118 individuals were assessed in three areas: occlusive, oral habits, and oral abnormalities. A dental history using a standardized form was taken from the primary care providers of all individuals.

Methods

All individuals were evaluated in the pediatric dental suite of the outpatient clinic of a pediatric hospital. Dental auxiliaries and pediatric nursing assistance was available on all patients. A pediatrician and a child psychologist were available for consultation. Examinations of the individuals were conducted while they were seated in a dental chair. The primary providers were interviewed, depending on age and individual circumstances. Dental photographs were obtained on all individuals. Panorex films and impressions were taken on selected individuals. Findings were recorded on a computerized data sheet. All individuals were evaluated by the same pedodontist.

Results

The individuals evaluated presented a high incidence of cranial and dental anomalies. Since these features usually affect the individual occlusion of the dentition, a large deviation in occlusal relationship was demonstrated by this group. Mesial occlusion, open-bite, and posterior cross-bite were the types of malocclusion characteristic of this group (Figure 5.2 A, B, C, D). A common

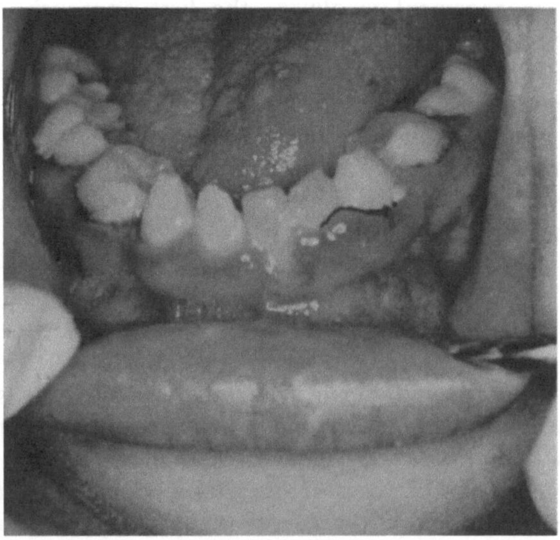

FIGURE 5.1. Individual with Down syndrome with plaque and gingivitis.

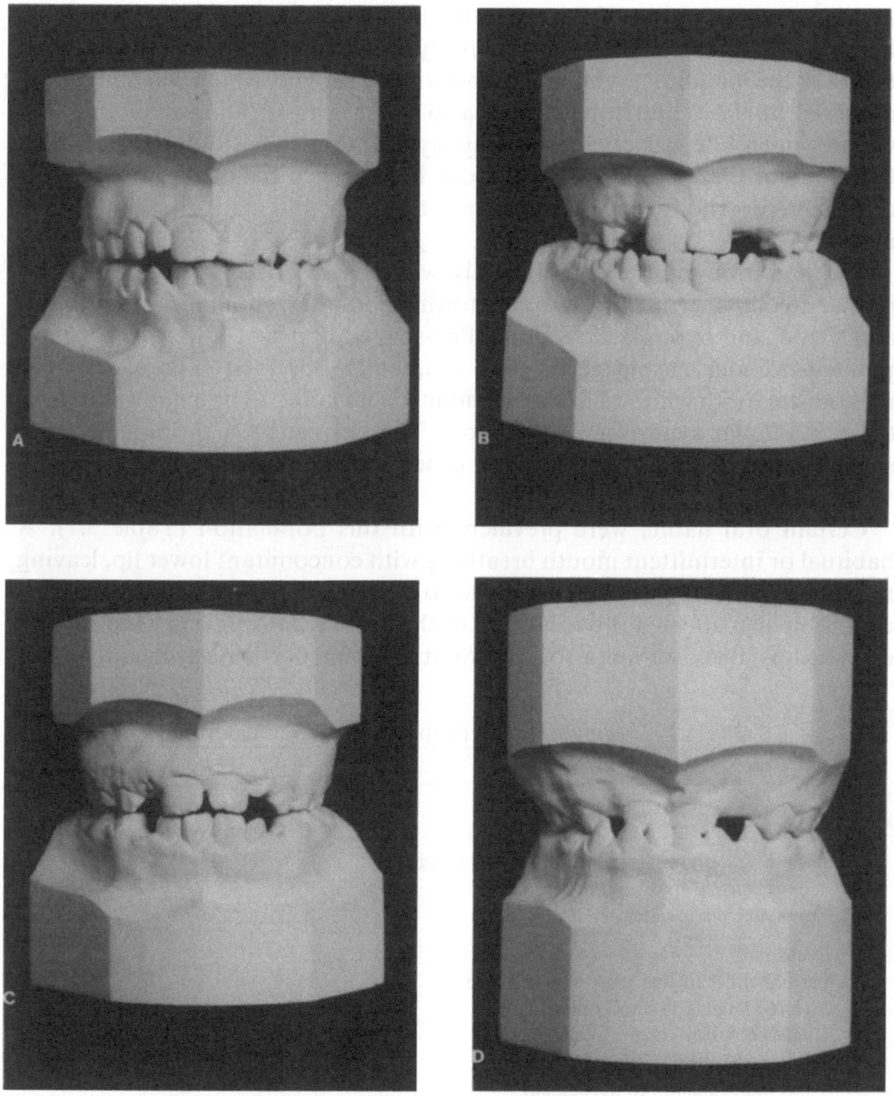

FIGURE 5.2A. Anterior malocclusion.
FIGURE 5.2B. Posterior cross–bite.
FIGURE 5.2C. Anterior open–bite.
FIGURE 5.2D. Anterior cross–bite.

finding was protrusion of the mandible in relation to the upper jaw, which may occur as a result of deficient maxillary growth and/or increased growth in length of the mandible. A large, low-positioned tongue, which was commonly observed in these individuals, may also cause a protruding mandible. An anterior open-bite was often caused by atypical tongue positions (Figure 5.2B, C). Many of these patients had a short, high-arched palate; the tongue was often seen protruding or resting between the teeth, and many times out of the mouth.

The dentition of these individuals was characterized by over-retained primary teeth, unerupted permanent teeth, anodontia, anomalies in tooth size and shape, and hypoplastic enamel. Peg-shaped upper or lower incisors and pointed, slender cuspid teeth were frequently observed (Figure 5.3). The mesiodistal tooth width of these individuals were noted to be narrower than in the non–Down syndrome population. The permanent dentition of these subjects may be said to display true generalized microdontia (Shafer et al., 1963).

Certain oral habits were prevalent with this population (Table 5.1). A habitual or intermittent mouth breathing with concomitant lower lip, leaving the mouth half open and the tongue to be seen, is frequently noted. This condition also affected the condition of the mouth, causing a dry mouth and cracked lips. Bruxism was also a common problem, particularly in individuals

TABLE 5.1. Common dental problems in Down syndrome.

		Percentage
Age range (infant to 19 years old)	188	(males: 90; females: 98)
Assuming individuals less than 2 years of age have normal findings and no teeth	70	
Total subjects in category reviewed	[118]	
Occlusion		
Permanent dentition with malocclusion (including cross-bites, open-bites, mesiocclusion, distocclusion)	15	13
Primary dentition with malocclusion	32	27
Total malocclusion in permanent and young dentition	47	40
Oral Habits		
Mouth breathing	99	84
Tongue thrusting	46	39
Digit sucking	42	36
Bruxism	50	42
Oral Abnormalities		
Caries	19	16
Bifid uvula	1	—
Geographic tongue	3	—
Furrowed tongue	65	55

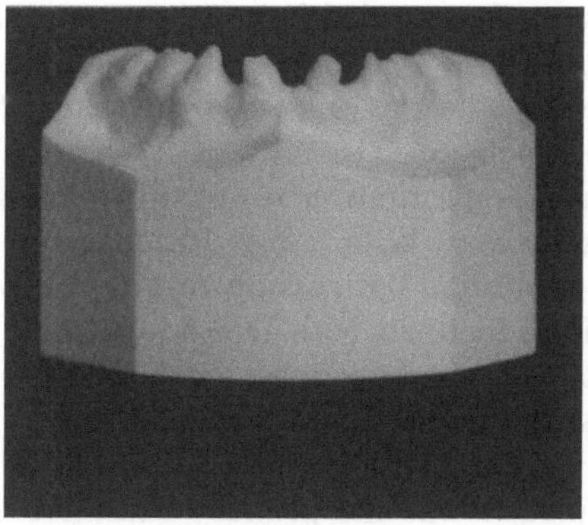

FIGURE 5.3. Peg-shaped lower incisor, pointed, cuspid teeth.

with lower cognitive function. Bruxism was noted in approximately 42% of this population (Table 5.1). Some other common dental problems, summarized in Table 5.1, were mouth breathing, tongue thrusting, and digit sucking.

Gingivitis was perhaps the most widespread oral problem evidenced by these individuals (Figure 5.1). Accumulations of food, plaque, and calculus produce inflammation of the gingiva and cause the tissues to become red, swollen, and hemorrhagic. The teeth most commonly affected by periodontal disease were the lower incisors, followed by the upper incisors and the upper and lower first permanent molars. The cuspids were generally the last teeth to be affected.

Discussion

The most common problems that differentiate the individual with Down syndrome from other patients include the physical disabilities that limit the patient's capacity to benefit from dental care, the patient's medical condition, communication problems, and the inability of the patient to adjust to novel circumstances. Anyone who has the opportunity to provide dental care to the person with Down syndrome will become aware of the problem of poor oral hygiene. It is not unusual to see cases in which oral hygiene has been totally neglected. Severe periodontal problems and needless loss of teeth is the usual result.

A restricted diet and abnormal muscular activity in the individual may add to the poor dental health evidenced by many of these individuals. It has been observed that children with more serious physical disabilities tend to eat a softer diet than other children with disabilities, perhaps due to a lack of oral muscular coordination. This, along with improper masticatory function and inadequate oral hygiene, is detrimental to the periodontal condition. Patients who are severely mentally retarded but without muscular impairment also have a tendency to consume soft foods with few detergent properties.

Patients must be shown how to practice proper oral hygiene. If they cannot demonstrate self-care, someone else must assist them. Chronic recurrence of gingival inflammation and irritation result in progressive gingivitis, which leads to periodontal disease. With a high incidence of poor oral hygiene, a greater degree of periodontal destruction results. Early bone destruction is often encountered in individuals with Down syndrome at an early age, and this can progress to extensive bone loss, tooth mobility, and tooth loss.

In a study of institutionalized and noninstitutionalized individuals with Down syndrome by Keyes, Bellock, and Jordan (1971), it was found that bacteria in dental plaque was the primary causative agent of periodontal disease in institutionalized Down syndrome individuals. They also observed that individuals who were free from dental plaque had no signs of periodontal problems. It has been observed by several investigators that periodontal disease begins at an early age in children with mental retardation, but there is general agreement that periodontal disease is most severe in individuals with Down syndrome (Cohen & Winer, 1965). Bacterial populations in the plaque of these patients were studied by Cutress, Brown, and Guy (1970). They found that the organisms in the bacterial flora of these individuals are different from those found in other individuals, for the bacterial organism bacteriodes melaninogenicus was found in greater concentrations. It has been speculated that there is a direct relationship between the presence of this bacteria and the incidence of periodontal disturbance. The incidence of dental caries in patients with Down syndrome has also been studied and has been found to be lower than in non–Down syndrome population. This may be due to various factors that range from the characteristics of salivary composition, lower salivary pH, and histologic and morphologic characteristics of the dentition.

Oral hygiene is very important for patients with Down syndrome. Hygiene aids such as battery-operated toothbrushes, water piks, and extended length, hand-held toothbrushes can be used for technical assistance. It is also recommended that these individuals have frequent dental visits for periodic teeth cleaning and dental evaluation. A regimen of good oral hygiene, use of dental rinses, proper diet, and regular visits to the dentists are the minimum care that an individual with Down syndrome should receive to maintain an oral condition free of chronic, destructive oral disease.

Common problems that differentiate the individual with this syndrome from other patients include medical conditions that can deter effective dental care, physical disabilities that can limit the patient's capacity to benefit from dental care, and absence of or limited motivation. Inability to adapt to essential routines or use prescribed appliances, and difficulties in communication arising from any cause, are barriers to dental hygiene. Sensitivity on the part of the dentist to the unique need of each patient is of prime importance. As pointed out earlier, these patients present with diverse medical, physical, and emotional problems, each of which can influence the choice of dental care.

Each patient should be evaluated on the basis of all the available information, including medical records. Many physicians will discuss a patient's condition over the telephone, but it is necessary to submit a release signed by the patient in order to obtain confidential information.

With the increased life expectancy of individuals with Down syndrome, the dental practitioner will come into contact with increasing numbers of these patients in his or her private office. Dental care for this population does not differ intrinsically from that of other patients. However, understanding the special needs of these individuals is a prerequisite to the provision of effective dental care.

Summary

Though individuals with Down syndrome have fewer dental caries than the general population, they have an increased incidence and frequency of gingivitis and resulting complications, including tooth loss. Common habits are bruxism, tongue thrusting, digit sucking, and mouth breathing. Malocclusion is seen in over 40% of these individuals. Children with Down syndrome need to see the dentist earlier and more frequently than other children, particularly if there is gingivitis. Oral hygiene needs to be aggressive, using oral hygiene aids. With behavioral management and the use of auxillaries, most individuals with Down syndrome can be treated in an out-patient setting.

References

Cohen, M.M., & Winer, R.A. (1965). Dental and facial characteristics in Down's syndrome (Mongolism). *Bulletin of the Academy of Dentally Handicapped, 3*(1), 18–27.

Cutress, T.W., Brown, R.H., & Guy, E.M. (1970). Occurrence of some bacterial species in the dental plaque of trisomy 21 (Mongoloid), other mentally retarded, and normal subjects. *New Zealand Dental Journal, 66*(304), 153–161.

Greenwood, R.D., & Nadus, A.S. (1976). The clinical course of cardiac disease in Down's syndrome. *Pediatrics*, (58P)6, 893–897.

Keyes, P.H., Bellock, G., & Jordan, H.V. (1971). Studies on the pathogenesis of destructive lesions of the gums and teeth in mentally retarded children. I. Dentobacterial plaque infection in children with Down's syndrome. *Clinical Pediatrics, 10*(12), 711–718.

Shafer, W.G., Hine, M.K., & Levy, B.M. (1963). *A textbook of oral pathology*, 2d ed. (p 35). Philadelphia: W.B. Sanders.

Smith, D.W. (1982). *Recognizable patterns of human malformation*. Philadelphia: W.B. Saunders.

6
Foot and Other Musculoskeletal Problems

CHERYL A. GAHAGEN AND DON C. VAN DYKE

Introduction

The majority of acquired orthopedic problems in persons with Down syndrome frequently result from joint hyperextensibility due to soft tissue laxity and muscular hypotonia. Goldberg and Ampola (1976) estimate that approximately 26% of this population demonstrate some orthopedic deformity. Reported deficits include atlantoaxial subluxation, scoliosis, spondylolisthesis, spina bifida occulta of the lumbar vertebrae, slipped capital femoral epiphyses, recurrent patellar dislocation with chondromalacia, pes planovalgus, and several forefoot deformities (Diamond et al., 1981; Goldberg & Ampola, 1976; Hreidarsson et al., 1982; Scheffler, 1973; Mahan et al., 1983; Van Dyke et al., 1988).

Neck

Atlantoaxial (C1/C2) subluxation has been reported by a number of authors in individuals with Down syndrome (Finerman, et al., 1976; Hreidarsson et al., 1982; Pueschel & Scola, 1987; Semine, et al., 1978). Its incidence is felt to be in the range of 10–20% with reports ranging from 9 to 31% (Martel & Tishler, 1966; Pueschel et al., 1981; Spitzer et al., 1961; Tishler & Martel, 1965). In those with radiographic evidence of C1/C2 subluxation (atlanto-dens interval $\geqslant 5$ mm), only 1.5% have been shown to be symptomatic, demonstrating neurological signs of spinal cord compression (Pueschel & Scola, 1987). Because of these concerns, the Committee on Sports Medicine of the American Academy of Pediatrics has recommended restrictions on sports activities that involve potential stress or trauma to the head and neck region, and lateral X-rays of the cervical spine to rule out C1/C2 subluxation (American Academy of Pediatrics, 1984). Some organizations, such as the Special Olympics, have placed specific prohibitions on training and competitive activities in Down syndrome individuals with C1/C2 instability (Special Olympics Bulletin, 1983). This has stimulated frequent discussion and commentaries in the literature (Pueschel, 1988; Van Dyke & Gahagen, 1988).

Back

Scoliosis may occur in up to 50% of individuals with Down syndrome. Curves are usually 20 degrees or less, and are equally distributed between left and right thoracic curves. Spinal curves appear to be related to soft tissue insufficiency and rarely progress. Bracing is infrequently required (Diamond et al., 1981).

Foot and Lower Extremities

Several authors have documented the occurrence of foot deformities in the individual with this syndrome (Diamond et al., 1981; Goldberg & Ampola, 1976; Mahan et al., 1983; Scheffler, 1973). There is, however, little discussion in the literature regarding medical management. Diamond et al. (1981) have described surgical intervention in specific cases. The foot types seen in Down syndrome are consistent with a flexible flat foot, with loss of longitudinal arch (Figures 6.1, 6.2, 6.3). In the absence of the longitudinal arch, body-weight

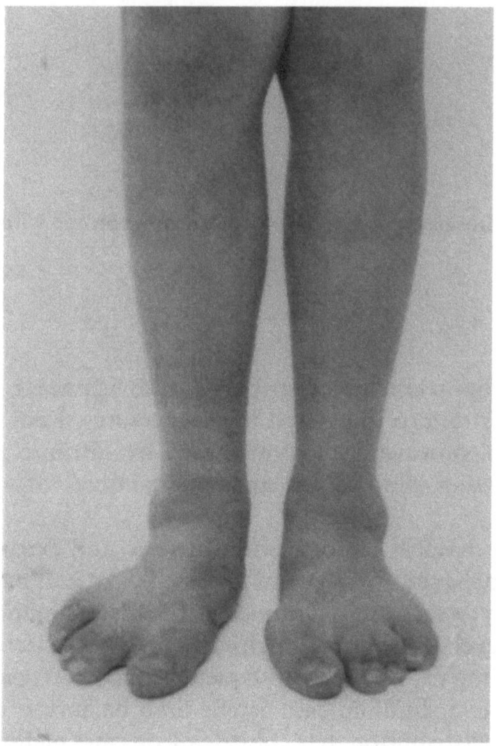

FIGURE 6.1. Fifteen-year-old male with Down syndrome with medial subtalor displacement, left greater than right; navicular weight bearing, lack of longitudinal arch; poor heel-toe alignment; subtalar misalignment with compensatory toe position.

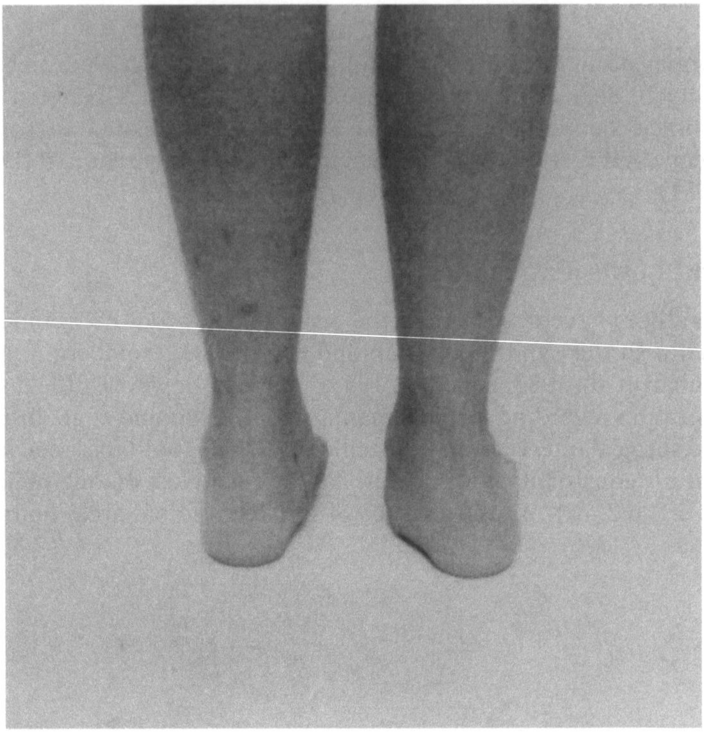

FIGURE 6.2. Fifteen-year-old male with Down syndrome with calcaneovalgus.

forces are disproportionately distributed and ligaments are overstressed, causing chronic strain to joints and joint structures. Foot posture in Down syndrome is not, however, solely mediated by intrinsic pronation forces. Femoral retroversion, genu valgus, and external tibial torsion also effect foot posture.

Altered biomechanical factors, both intrinsic and extrinsic to the Down syndrome foot, produce an awkward and inefficient gait pattern. It also may be influenced by weak or hypotonic gatro-soleus complex or be due to developmental level. The absent longitudinal arch, the decreased work of the plantar flexor complex, and the subsequent reduced vertical displacement of the body promote a shuffling gait. Single limb balance is precarious due to improper weight distribution over the calcaneous and metatarsals. Therefore, step width is often increased to widen the base of support, creating a wide-based gait that is not uncommon in the individual with Down syndrome. Upper body rotation is frequently limited, and arm swing is reduced.

Forefoot deformities appear to be extremely common in the adolescent and adult with Down syndrome (Figures 6.1, 6.2). The most common deformities, metatarsus primus varus with hallux varus or hallux valgus, appear related to the hypermobility of the first ray. Lateral displacement of the great toe may force lateral displacement of the remaining toes, causing toe crowding and overlapping (Figure 6.1). Toe alignment is often inherently compromised by such primary anomalies as metatarsal shortening and syndactyly. The wide interspace between the first and second toe (Goldstein's sign) is caused by adduction of the first metatarsal. As the individual ages, chronic foot deformities often become symptomatic. Progressive disfigurement makes shoe wear uncomfortable; foot pain limits ambulation. Subtalar instability results in deviant distribution, poor limb posture, awkward gait, and deficient balance skills. Although subtalar instability is often corrected by orthotic intervention in the normal population, treatment of subtalar instability in the population with Down syndrome does not routinely occur.

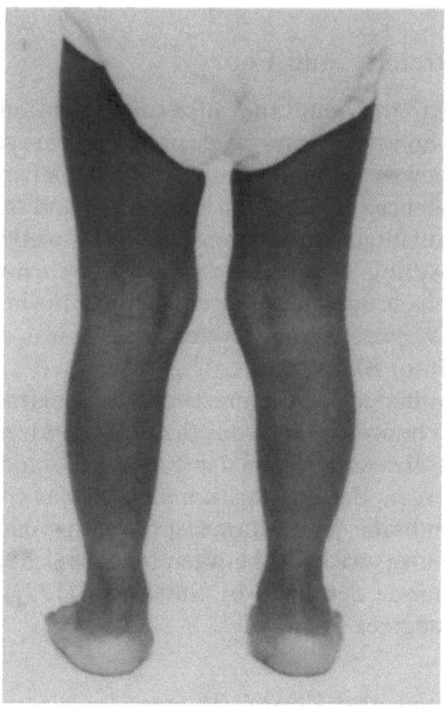

FIGURE 6.3. Thirty-month-old male with Down syndrome without orthosis. Note differences between young versus older child (e.g., soft tissue changes and bony remodeling).

Methods and Patient Population

Subgroups of Patient Population

Of the 190 individuals with Down syndrome (described in the Introduction and Appendix I), four subgroups were studied. The four areas of investigation were cervical spine abnormalities, back problems, foot abnormalities, and the use of orthoses in Down syndrome children with foot abnormalities.

Neck

X-rays of the cervical spine region of 34 Down individuals older than 5 years of age were obtained and reviewed for C1/C2 subluxation. A developmental age of 5 years was selected for radiographs because at this age individuals were able to cooperate to obtain a technically satisfactory study (Van Dyke & Gahagen, 1988). Radiographs demonstrating 5 mm or greater distance between C1 and C2 were given the diagnosis of atlantoaxial instability. In addition, cervical spine films of 12 adult Down syndrome individuals were reviewed retrospectively.

Back, Lower Extremity, and Foot

The back, lower extremity, and foot of a subpopulation of 67 children with Down syndrome who were 3 years of age or older were evaluated by a physical therapist and reviewed by a developmental pediatrician. The back was examined for evidence of lordosis, kyphosis, and scoliosis. Data were analyzed on 67 individuals as children walked on walking boards and on a hardwood floor covering. Detailed examinations were not possible in all cases due to lack of patient cooperation. Extensibility of the hips, knees, and ankles were evaluated. Assessment of gross motor skills was determined using the Peabody Gross Motor Skills test.

The foot was evaluated for the presence of a longitudinal arch. This was done by having children stand on the floor and making a subjective assessment of the absence, minimal presence, or moderate presence of a longitudinal arch. A moderate longitudinal arch was considered the normal arch pattern. The subtalar joint was measured with goniometer. Upon weight bearing, the angle measured was between the Achilles tendon and a vertical upright by a technique described by Subotnick (1979). The greatest angle measured was 15 degrees.

Foot Abnormalities and Foot Orthoses

Orthoses were made for those individuals with foot problems, primarily, absent longitudinal arch. The orthoses were made by an orthotist from a plaster cast obtained with a subtalar joint firmly held in a nonweight-bearing

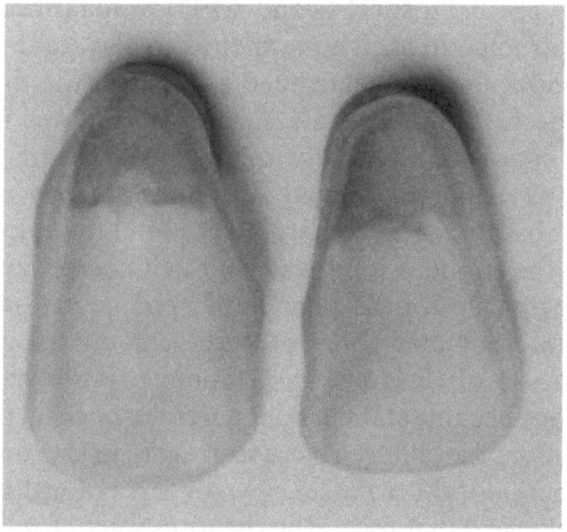

FIGURE 6.4. Foot orthoses.

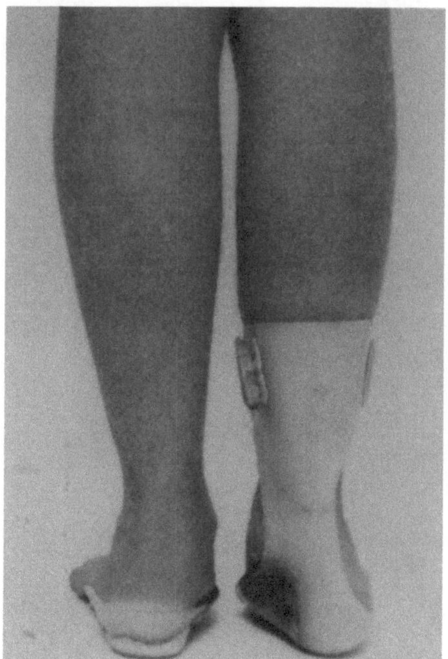

FIGURE 6.5. Fifteen-year-old male with Down syndrome with foot orthoses.

neutral position. The orthoses (FO and AFO) were fabricated from polypropylene, and constructed in such a manner as to elevate the longitudinal arch with the apex under the navicular head and extending distally to terminate proximally to the first three metatarsal heads (Figures 6.4, 6.5). The arch support tapered laterally and distally to prevent elevations of the foot's lateral border. Medial navicular placement was prevented by a high medial wall (Figure 6.5). The orthoses was constructed to hold the calcaneous in a neutral position so that the subtalar joint was held in a correct anatomical position, determined by palpation of the talar head. The neutral position of balance between the hind foot and forefoot was achieved (Figures 6.5, 6.6). As abnormal pronation of the foot was eliminated and the longitudinal arch supported, the foot became stable under a weight-bearing position. Following the initial evaluation, the children were seen again in two or three weeks for assessment of proper fit of the orthoses. Two or three months later, they were reevaluated by a physical therapist. The orthoses were checked and the parents were questioned.

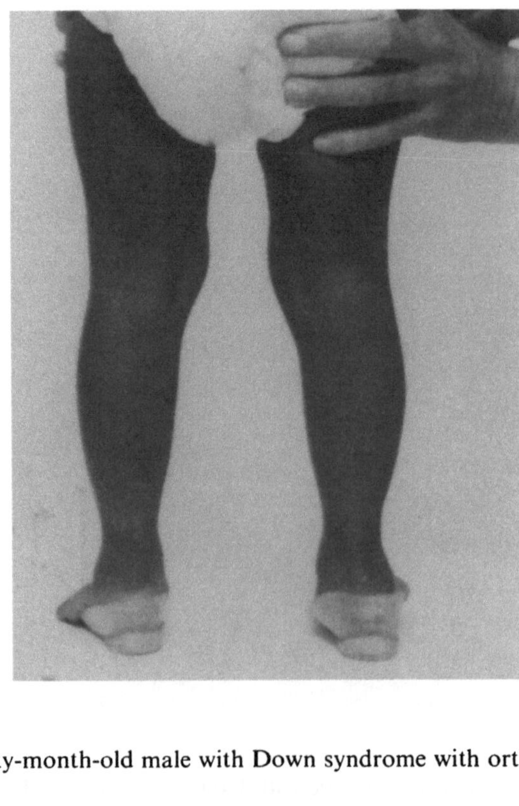

FIGURE 6.6. Thirty-month-old male with Down syndrome with orthosis (same child as Figure 6.3)

Results

Neck

Of 34 Down syndrome individuals in the study between the ages of 5 and 21 years, 3 of 34 (9%) demonstrated 5 mm or greater distance between C1/C2 subluxation and were given the diagnosis of atlantoaxial instability (Table 6.1) (Van Dyke & Gahagen, 1988). Review of the cervical spine in adult individuals 26 to 42 years of age showed degenerative changes of the cervical spine with no evidence of C1/C2 subluxation (Table 6.2).

TABLE 6.1. Atlantoaxial instability in Down syndrome.

Patient number	Age (yrs)	Gender	Radiographic finding
1	10	Male	C1/C2 subluxation (5 mm)
2	17	Male	C1/C2 subluxation (6 mm)
3	12	Male	C1/C2 subluxation (>5 mm)

Number of patients receiving radiograph of the cervical region to r/o C1/C2 subluxation = 34. Number of positive cervical radiographs for C1/C2 subluxation = 3.
Source: Van Dyke et al., 1988

TABLE 6.2. Radiographs of cervical spine in adults with Down syndrome.

Patient number	Age (yrs)	Gender	Findings
4	42	Male	Mild to moderate degenerative spurring throughout the cervical spine; mild to moderate narrowing of the right C4/C5 neuroforamine; possible mild narrowing of left C3/C4 neuroforamine
5	33	Male	Moderate degenerative changes with disc space narrowing and anterior osteophytes; minor posterior osteophytes
6	32	Male	Degenerative spondylosis with narrowing of the C5/C6 disc interspace and moderate hypertrophic osteoarthritic marginal osteophyte formation around narrowed interspace, projecting posteriorly into the right neura foramen causing some encroachment on space C5/C6
7	26	Female	Mild degenerative arthritis with anterior spur formation at C5/C6

Source: Van Dyke et al., 1988

Back, Lower Extremity, and Foot

Scoliosis in 11% and lordosis in 14% were the most common back abnormalities (Table 6.3). The initial examination of the lower extremity in a Down population of 67 individuals showed that 28% (19) had a compensative gait, 10% (7) had a very young or primitive gait, and the remainder had a normal gait pattern. Examination of the strength in the various muscle groups of the lower extremities showed inadequate strength in only 8% (5). On evaluation of range and motion of the hips, knees, and ankles, 40% (27) had minimal hyperextensibility, with 26% (17) demonstrated a moderate degree of hyperextensibility of one or more joints (Table 6.3).

Evaluation of the foot of those children with Down syndrome who cooperated showed that only 8% of this population had a normal longitudinal arch. Forty-two percent (22) had a minimal arch, and the same number had no longitudinal arch. Measuring of the subtalar joints showed that there was a significant degree of calcaneovalgus, greater than 5 degrees in 46% (27) of the 59 individuals in which this joint angle could be measured.

Foot Abnormalities and Orthoses

An evaluation of orthoses at two to three months post-initial fitting of the orthoses showed that total correction of the hind foot alignment was

TABLE 6.3. Musculoskeletal problems in persons with Down syndrome (3–18 years of age).[a]

Problem	N		%
Back Alignment (abnormalities)			
(66)			
1 Lordosis	9		14
2 Kyphosis	3		5
3 Lordosis/kyphosis	2		3
4 Lordosis/kyphosis/scoliosis	5		
5 Lordosis/scoliosis	1	(7)	11[a]
6 Scoliosis	1		
Lower Extremity (assessment of function)			
Gait			
Primitive gait	7		10
(67) Compensatory	19		28
Range of motion of hip, knee, ankle			
(67) Minimal hyperextensibility	27		40
Moderate hyperextensibility	17		26
Foot			
Longitudinal arch			
(53) Absent	22		42
Minimal	22		42
Moderate (normal)	4		8
Subtalar joint			
(59) Calcaneovalgus	27		46

[a]Summation of: 4,5,6

commonly not achieved. Goniometric measurements of the foot demonstrated, however, that calcaneovalgus in all cases was reduced by at least 50% or more. In general, the age of the child was in inverse proportion to the degree of observed functional improvement. In all age groups, consistent use of foot orthoses appeared to improve foot and limb posture when the orthoses were worn (Figures 6.5, 6.6). When the calcaneovalgus was directed from valgus to a position under the talus, the forefoot returned from abduction and the toes assumed a forward direct position. In addition, the knees were redirected and the hips derotated centering over the knees and ankles. Orthotic control of the subtalar joint helped minimize specific gait deficiencies and decreased the degree of out-toeing.

Parental responses were also recorded regarding the child's ambulation, balance, and developmental skills. Parents of young ambulators indicated that their children appeared more competent after an initial one to two weeks of adjustment when the orthoses were worn. Parents indicated the incidence of stumbling and falling decreased. They felt that ambulation velocity increased and that new skills such as running or walking backward were initiated. In the majority of cases, the parents noted significant improvement in ambulation and balance skills. Three individuals required modification of their orthoses because of skimprovement. In all age groups, consistent use of foot orthoses appeared to improve foot and limb posture when the orthoses were worn (Figures 6.5 and 6.6). When the calcaneovalgus was was directed from valgus to a position under the talus, the forefoot returned from abduction and the toes assumed a forward direct position. In addition, the knees were redirected and the hips derotated centering over the knees and ankles. Orthotic control of the subtalar joint helped minimize specific gait deficiencies and decreased the degree of out-toeing.

Parental responses were also recorded regarding the child's ambulation, balance, and developmental skills. Parents of young ambulators indicated that their children appeared more competent after an initial one to two weeks of adjustment when the orthoses were worn. Parents indicated the incidence of stumbling and falling decreased. They felt that ambulation velocity increased and that new skills such as running or walking backward were initiated. In the majority of cases, the parents noted significant improvement in ambulation and balance skills. Three individuals required modification of their orthoses because of skin breakdown under the navicular head. Another individual complained of excessive pain under the metatarsal head. In each case, modification of the orthoses corrected the problem.

Discussion

The incidence of atlantoaxial subluxation in this population was approximately 9% (Van Dyke & Gahagen, 1988). This is in general agreement with previous reported ranges of 10–20% (Hreidasson et al., 1982; Pueschel, 1983; Pueschel & Scola, 1987; Semine et al., 1978; Whaley & Gray, 1980). A prospective review of the cervical spine and radiographs of adults with Down syndrome showed no subluxation but significant degenerative changes of the cervical spine, with spur formation, narrowing of the foramena, narrowing of the disk inner space, and osteophyte formation (Van Dyke & Gahagen, 1988). Fidone (1986) in a study of 41 adult Down syndrome individuals had a similar finding with 16 of these individuals demonstrating varying degrees of degenerative arthritis of the cervical vertebrae and inner vertebral disk. Baseline radiographic studies of the cervical spine are indicated in all children older than 5 years (American Academy of Pediatrics, 1984; Pueschel et al., 1987; Van Dyke & Gahagen, 1988). X-rays should be a consideration on all Down syndrome adults, particularly those 30 years of age and older because of the significant findings of degenerative changes (Van Dyke & Gahagen, 1988; Fidone et al., 1986).

Scoliosis and lordosis were the most common back abnormalities noted in this population. There was no history of bracing being required. Examination of the lower extremities showed an absent longitudinal arch in calcaneal valgus with subtalar instability to be a frequent finding in Down syndrome individuals. Ankle instability was most pronounced in the young child, due to the presence of moderate to severe hypotonicity and ligamatous laxity. Soft tissue laxity appears to become lessened with increasing age and the ankle is inherently more stable in the older child.

Clinical observation suggests that the use of foot orthoses by individuals with Down syndrome improves gait patterns and balance skills. Down syndrome children appeared to easily adapt to orthoses and functional improvement was noted within two weeks of their use. Parents felt that the incidence of stumbling and falling decreased, while ambulation velocity increased, and new skills were initiated. Complaints and complications of the use of orthoses appear to be minimal. It is felt that a long-term controlled study is needed, matching age, sex, and developmental level with measurements and gait analysis to substantiate initial clinical observations for the use of such orthotic devices in Down syndrome individuals.

Summary

C1/C2 subluxation is seen in 10 to 20% of individuals with Down syndrome. Because of the potentially life-threatening complication of spinal cord compression, radiographic screening of Down syndrome individuals is warranted with appropriate precautions and follow-up for those individuals with radiographic findings. Degenerative changes are a frequent finding in the adult Down syndrome individual and X-rays need to be considered for this population, particularly if there are complaints of neck pain, limitations of motion, or neurologic findings.

Scoliosis and lordosis is not an uncommon clinical finding in the Down syndrome individual. However, progression is rare and bracing is infrequent.

Foot deformities appear to be a common finding in individuals, primarily the absence of a longitudinal arch and calcaneovalgus deformity. Preliminary clinical studies of foot orthoses in individuals with foot problems suggest that such orthotic intervention may be helpful in such individuals. Further studies need to occur.

References

American Academy of Pediatrics, Committee on Sports Medicine. (1984). Atlantoaxial instability in Down syndrome. *Pediatrics, 74*, 152–154.

Cailliet, R. (1983). *Foot and ankle pain*. Philadelphia: F.A. Davis Co.

Diamond, L.S., Lynne, D., & Sigman, B. (1981). Orthopedic disorders in patients with Down's syndrome. *Orthopedic Clinics of North America, 12* (1), 57–71.

Fidone, G.S. (1986). Degenerative cervical arthritis in Down syndrome. *N. Engl. J. Med., 312* (5), 320.

Finerman, G.A.M., Sakai, D., & Weingarten, S. (1976). Atlantoaxial dislocation with spinal cord depression in a Mongolian child: A case report. *Journal of Bone and Joint Surgery of America, 58*, 408–409.

Goldberg, M.J., & Ampola, M.G. (1976). Birth defect syndromes in which orthopedic problems may be overlooked. *Orthopedic Clinics of North America, 7* (2), 285.

Hreidarsson, S., Magram, G., & Singer, H. (1982). Symptomatic atlantoaxial dislocation in Down syndrome. *Pediatrics, 69* (5), 568–571.

Mahan, K.T., Diamond, E., & Brown, D. (1983). Podiatric profile of the Down's syndrome individual. *Journal of the American Psychological Association, 73* (4), 173–179.

Martel, W., & Tishler, J.M. (1966). Observations on the spine in Mongolism. *American Journal of Roentgenology Radium Thermal Nuclear Medicine, 94*, 630–638.

Pueschel, S.M. (1983). Atlantoaxial subluxation in Down syndrome. *Lancet, 1*, 980.

Pueschel, S.M. (1988). Atlantoaxial instability in Down syndrome. *Pediatrics, 81*(6), 879–880.

Pueschel, S.M., & Scola, F.H. (1987). Epidemiologic, radiographic, and clinical studies of atlantoaxial instability in individuals with Down syndrome. *Pediatrics, 80*, 555–560.

Pueschel, S.M., et al. (1981). Atlantoaxial instability in children with Down syndrome. *Pediatric Radiology, 10*, 129–132.

Scheffler, N.M. (1973). Down's syndrome and clinical findings related to the foot. *Journal of the American Psychological Association, 63* (1), 18–21.

Semine, A.A., Ertel, A.N., Goldberg, J.M., & Bull, M.J. (1978). Cervical spine instability: Children with Down syndrome (trisomy 21). *Journal of Bone and Joint Surgery of America, 60A*, 649–652.

Special Olympics Bulletin (1983). Participation by individuals with Down syndrome who suffer from atlantoaxial dislocation. Washington D.C.: Special Olympics, Inc.

Spitzer, R., Rabinowich, J.Y., & Wyber, K.C. (1961). A study of abnormalities of the skull, teeth, and lenses in Mongolis. *Canadian Medical Association Journal, 84*, 567–572.

Subotnick, S.I. (1979). *Cures for common running injuries*. Mountain View, Calif.: Anderson World Publishers.

Tishler, J.M., & Martel, W. (1965). Dislocation of the atlas in Mongolism: Preliminary report. *Radiology, 84*, 904–906.

Van Dyke, D.C., & Gahagan, C.A. (1988). Cervical spine abnormalities and problems in individuals with Down syndrome. *Clinical Pediatrics, 27* (9), 415–418.

Whaley, M.J., & Gray, W.D. (1980). Atlantoaxial dislocation in Down syndrome. *Canadian Medical Association Journal*, 123, 35–37.

7
Motor and Hand Function

MARTY NOVAK HOFFMAN, LINDA LUSARDI PETERSON,
AND DON C. VAN DYKE

Introduction

The frequency of soft-tissue laxity and gross and fine motor dysfunction makes it a common finding in occupational and physical therapy evaluations in programs dealing with older adults and young children with Down syndrome. In children with Down syndrome, hypotonia, increased flexibility of the joints, decreased muscle strength, and the frequent occurrence of significant congenital heart disease all contribute to potential motor delays in infancy and early childhood (Zausmer & Shea, 1984). Carr (1975) showed a severe deceleration in the rate of mental and motor development during the first two years of life in these children. The most significant declines in development occurred in the first 10 months. Delays in motor development appeared to occur more rapidly than those of mental development (Carr, 1975). In the child with Down syndrome, the generalized low muscle tone that contributes to motor delays has also been correlated with delayed speech acquisition, delayed cognitive development, impaired stereognosis, slower reaction time, and decreased kinesthetic feedback (Harris, 1984).

Zausmer and Shea (1984) studied 89 children with Down syndrome in a motor development program. Children from birth to three years were assessed periodically, focusing on muscle strength, range of motion, muscle tone, and developmental attainment. It was found that there were greater delays in gross motor skills than in grasp and prehension skills, with delays in all areas of gross and fine motor development. Those with moderate and severe congenital heart disease were more delayed in gross motor skills than those who had only mild heart problems. The results further showed that Down syndrome children in the program performed better when they were female, had no or minimal heart defects, had good muscle tone, and had adequate followthrough by parents (Schnell, 1984). In a study by Harris (1983) examining sex differences in mental and motor developmental in 20 children with Down syndrome, ages 2.7 months to 21.5 months, no significant differences were shown between males and females. In previous studies, however, it has been determined that females performed better than male Down syndrome children (LaVeck & LaVeck, 1977).

In a study by LaVeck and LaVeck (1977) of 40 children with Down syndrome, ages 12 to 36 months, using the Bayley Scales of Infant Development, the mental raw scores of males and females were found not to differ significantly. However, a significant difference did exist between motor scores of males and females. Clinical studies have consistently demonstrated a deceleration in the rate of mental and motor development with increasing chronological age and a consistent superiority of mental performance over motor performance (Harris, 1981; LaVeck & LaVeck, 1977).

In this study, the grip strength of 474 non-Down syndrome children between the ages of 5 and 12 years was used for comparison with the Down syndrome children (within that chronological age range) (Ager, Olivett, & Johnson, 1984). Studies have shown that in non-Down syndrome children, males scored significantly stronger in grip strength than females. Grip strength increased with chronological age. This study further ascertained that hand dominance is not a significant predictor of hand strength (Ager et al., 1984; Mathiowetz et al., 1986). One study that compared a control group (N = 33) of normal children to a study group (N = 28) of children with Down syndrome concluded that the children with Down syndrome showed increases in grip strength with increases in age (Morris, Vaughan, & Vaccano, 1982). However, there was a significant difference in the grip strength between the controls and the children with Down syndrome; the controls were stronger ($p < 0.05$) (Morris et al., 1982).

Population

Subgroups of the Down syndrome population described in the Introduction and Appendix I were studied to assess gross motor development, fine motor development, and hand function (Table 7.1). Hand function was studied in detail from the perspective of dominance, grip strength, pencil grasp and pincer grasp. The assessment form used appears in Table 7.2.

TABLE 7.1. Down patient population evaluated.

Test	Males	Females	Total[a]	Cardiac[a]	Age (yrs)	Mean age (yrs)
PFM	74	75	149	58	0.1–19.1	3.6
PF and GM	30	30	60	21	2.5–19.0	7.3
McC and GM	26	23	49	14	3.8–19.0	10.1
BMS	41	51	92	41	0.1–9.1	1.4
BM and MS	38	46	86	38	1.0–9.1	1.7

[a]Cardiac = any evidence of significant cardiac disease by examination and/or history.
Note: PFM = Peabody Fine Motor; PF and GM = Peabody Fine and Gross Motor; McCF and GM = McCarthy Fine and Gross Motor; BMS = Bayley Motor Scale; and BM and MS = Bayley Mental and Motor Scale.

TABLE 7.2. Assessment of motor and hand functions.

Gross and fine motor assessment

Motor maturity

1) Movement assessment of infants (birth–1 year)

	Risk Score
Muscle tone:	________
Primitive reflexes:	________
Automatic reactions:	________
Volitional movement:	________
Total risk score:	________

2) Bayley motor Scales (birth–30 months):
   Raw score ________ Development level ________
3) Peabody developmental—fine motor (birth–83 months):
   Raw score ________ Development level ________
4) McCarthy scales of children's abilities ($2\frac{1}{2}$–$8\frac{1}{2}$ yrs):
   Fine motor ________ Total (OT/PT) raw score ________
   Overall motor level ________
5) Bruininks-Osterestsky test of motor proficiency ($4\frac{1}{2}$–$14\frac{1}{2}$ yrs):
   Raw score ________ Developmental level ________

Hand Function

1) Grip strength (3 yrs–adult):

Right: ———	Total: ____	Average: ____	Average for age: ____
Left: ———	Total: ____	Average: ____	Average for age: ____

2) Dominance:

a) Hand:	Right	Left	Undecided
b) Eye:	Right	Left	Undecided
c) Foot:	Right	Left	Undecided

3) Hand use:

a) Hand grip of crayon/pencil	Right	Left	Both
____ Palmar supinate			
____ Digital prinate			
____ Static tripod			
____ Dynamic tripod			
b) Grasp of cube:	Right	Left	Both
____ Palmar grasp			
____ Radial palmar			
____ Radial digital			
c) Grasp of pellet:	Right	Left	Both
____ Raking			
____ Scissor			
____ Inferior pincer			
____ Neat pincer			
d) Hand structure:	Typical		Atypical
e) Crossing Midline:			
(at least 3 out of 4)			Time
Pennies:	yes	no	____ sec
Stack cones:	yes	no	____ sec
Sorting box:	yes	no	____ sec
Stack blocks:	yes	no	____ sec
f) Nine hole peg test:	________________		
g) Reaction time:	Slow	Average	Rapid

(*Continued on p. 96*)

TABLE 7.2. (*Cont.*)

Gross and fine motor assessment		
Upper Extremity		
1) Muscle tone:		
Hypotonic	Slightly hypotonic	Normal
2) Passivity (wrists):		
Does not tighten	Many flaps then tighten	Few flaps then tighten
3) Consistency (biceps and triceps):		
Soft with little resistance	In between	Muscle sturdy
4) Range of motion:		
Wrist:	Right ________	Left ________
Hyperextensible	Normal	Tight
Elbow:	Right ________	Left ________
Hyperextensible	Normal	Tight

Source: Linda Lusardi Peterson, 1984.

Methods

Motor Assessment

A portion of the evaluation consisted of assessment of gross motor development using the Bayley Scale of Infant Development (BSID), the Peabody Developmental Motor Scale (PDMS), and the motor portion of the McCarthy Scale of Cognitive Assessment (MSCA). Some children were tested using more than one of these tools (Table 7.1).

Eighty-six children were assessed using the BSID (mental and motor scales): 38 males, 46 females, and two of undetermined sex. Their ages ranged from 0.1 to 9.1 years with a mean age of 1.7 years (only five children over 6 years were tested). Thirty-eight had some cardiac involvement ranging from insignificant to moderately severe. On the PDMS (fine and gross motor), 60 children (30 males and 30 females) were tested for both gross and fine motor skills. Their ages ranged from 2.5 to 19 years, with a mean age of 7.3 years. Twenty-one had reported cardiac problems. On the MSCA, 49 children were assessed: 26 males and 23 females. Ages ranged from 3.8 to 19.0 years, with a mean age of 10.1 years. Fourteen had reported cardiac problems.

The history for fine motor development of a total of 178 children (with an age range 0.1–19.1 years) was reviewed by an occupational therapist. All children were living at home. Seventy-seven of the children assessed had some type of cardiac history. Parents identified whether their child had therapy (occupational, physical, or speech) prior to evaluation. Out of the total of 190 children seen in the program, 154 (81%) had received some form of therapy, either alone or in a combination.

To assess motor performance, the BSID, MSCA, and PDMS were used as part of the evaluation. Depending on the chronological and developmental

TABLE 7.3. Grip strength, hand dominance, and grasp.

Area evaluated	Males	Females	Total	Age (yrs)	Mean age (yrs)
Grip strength	26	24	50	4.2–19.9	10.3
Hand dominance	—	—	67	4.2–19.0	10.3
Pencil grasp	—	—	107	1.0–19.0	—
Pincer grasp	—	—	109	5.0–12.0	—

age, the Movement Assessment Scale for Infants and the Bruininks-Osteretsky Test of Motor Proficiency were also used.

Assessment of Hand Function

Hand function was defined as grip strength in bilateral hands, hand dominance, type of grasp of a pencil, and type of pincer grasp of a small object (pellet) (Table 7.2). Grip strength was observed in 50 children (26 males, 24 females) (Table 7.3). Ages of the children were 4.2 to 19.9 years with a mean age of 10.3 years. A Jammar dynamometer was used, with each hand tested three times. Children switched hands between readings, and short rest periods (10–20 seconds) were given between each reading.

Hand dominance was also identified in 67 of the children. However, only 39 children were tested for both grip strength and hand dominance. Hand dominance was defined in the screening program as that hand which children most frequently used to spontaneously pick up a variety of objects.

Types of pencil grasp were observed in 107 children tested between the ages of 1 and 19 years. The types of grasp of a pencil were taken from Erhardt Developmental Prehension Assessment, which identified four grasps, changing with developmental age (Erhardt, 1982).

One-hundred nine of the children tested were identified for pincer grasp. Types of pincer were taken from the PDMS (fine motor) and included: (1) raking or scraping fingers along surface to secure object into palm; (2) inferior pincer—opposition of pad of thumb to lateral side of index finger; and (3) superior pincer—opposition of pad of thumb to pad of index fingers. Ages tested were from 5 months to 12 years. All children seen beyond this age had a superior pincer grasp.

Results

Gross Motor and Fine Motor Development

Gross motor skills exceeded fine motor skills. We found this to be true with the children tested on the Peabody Fine and Gross Motor Scales. Of the 60 children (0.1–19.1 years of age) tested, 4 had the same score for both gross and fine motor, 20 tested higher in fine motor, and 36 tested higher in gross motor (Table 7.4).

TABLE 7.4. Gross motor, fine motor, and mental function.

Item	Number
Test: Peabody (gross and fine motor); N = 60.	
Gross motor = fine motor	4
Gross motor greater than fine motor	36
Gross motor less than fine motor	20
Total	60
Test: Bayley (mental and motor); N = 86	
Mental function = motor function	19
Mental function greater than motor function	52
Mental function less than motor function	15
Total	86

Using the Mann-Whitney-Wilcoxon sum rank test, 60% of the children were found to exceed in gross motor skills ($p < 0.05$) in comparison to their fine motor development. Males performed significantly better on gross motor skills than females ($p < 0.05$). There was no significant difference between gross and fine motor performance in females. Children without cardiac involvement did not show a statistically significant difference in performance between gross and fine motor skills, whereas those with cardiac problems did show a significant difference ($p < 0.05$).

On the BSID, children with Down syndrome show a decrease in mental and motor development when compared to normal children. However, mental performance was consistently higher than motor performance in males and females regardless of cardiac involvement. In our study, 86 children were tested using both the BSID mental and motor scales. Nineteen children had the same scores on the mental and motor scales; 15 had higher motor scores and 52 had higher mental scores (Table 7.4). Children tested on the BSID showed that 66% had higher mental scores compared to motor scores, even though an overall deceleration was noted in both areas. We did not find any statistically significant difference between males and females on either the mental or motor portion of the BSID, contrary to some previously reported literature (LaVeck & LaVeck, 1977) (Carr, 1975). Our findings are in agreement with much of the available data concerning development of children with Down syndrome.

Hand Function and Grip Strength

The grip strength of Down syndrome females in our study showed much wider variability in their scores than did the males. However, this observation was not statistically supported once controlled for age. Our testing supported the previous study by Morris et al. (1982), which showed that grip strength of children with Down syndrome was significantly lower than that of normal children.

TABLE 7.5. Grasp of a pencil.

Palmar-supinate: The average age range for attaining a palmar supinate grasp was between 13 and 36 months.
Norm (1-2 yrs)[a]
Digital-pronate: The average age range for attaing a digital-pronate grasp was between 24 months and 5 years.
Norm (2-3 yrs)[a]
Static tripod: The average age range for attaining a static tripod grasp was between 4 and 8 years.
Norm (3-4 yrs)[a]
Dynamic tripod: The average age range for attaining a dynamic tripod grasp was between 5 and 12 years.
Norm (4-6 yrs)[a]
Grasp of a Pellet
Raking: The average age range was between 7 months and 2 yrs.
Inferior pincer: The average age range was between 15 months and 3.5 yrs.
Superior pincer: The average age range was between 18 months and 4 yrs.

[a]Norms from Erhardt, Developmental Hand Dysfunction, 1982.

There were no significant differences noted between males and females on either right-or left-handed scores for grip strength, even when corrected for age. There was also no difference in the left-hand grip strength scores of the left-hand-dominant children when compared to the left-hand grip strength scores of right-hand-dominant children. There was no statistical significance in the right grip strength scores of the left-hand-dominant children compared to the right grip strength scores of the right-hand-dominant ones.

Grasp

To identify age of attainment in grasp of a pencil and grasp of a pellet, an average range was used, as statistical analysis could not be completed due to variability in the ages and scores (Table 7.5).

Hand Dominance

Hand dominance was identified in 67 children. Forty-nine (73%) were identified as right-hand dominant; 18 (27%) were identified as left-hand dominant (Table 7.3).

Discussion

Gross motor skills exceeded fine motor skills in males with Down syndrome, but not in females. Cardiac involvement had a significant effect on gross and fine motor performance. Down syndrome children, with time, showed a decline in mental and motor development, but cognitive performance in both sexes was consistently higher than motor performance, even when there was cardiac involvement.

Hand dominance was not a statistically significant predictor of hand strength for the left or right hand. Although statistical analysis was not used to verify the information in the pencil and small-objects grasps, it was the authors' opinion that this information, as it is cited in age ranges, could be beneficial in a clinical treatment setting (Table 7.5). Grip of a pencil and small object showed that children in the sample generally followed the same sequence as those outlined by Erhardt and from the PDMS. Differences existed in the length of time of attainment, with the children with Down syndrome showing wider variability. Further research is indicated in this area.

The age ranges at which various grasping patterns occur indicate that with increasing age there is wider variability in attainment of these skills. This wide variability among mastery of hand function skills in children with Down syndrome is consistent with the wide variability in overall attainment of motor skills. Some early skills (palmar-supinate and digital-pronate grasp) were beginning to emerge at generally the same time as in other children.

Our findings both differed from and supported the cited studies in grip strength. Of interest was the high variability in female scores. Males with Down syndrome did not score statistically higher than females, a finding that contradicts previous research in this area for normal children (Ager et al., 1984).

Summary

Gross motor skills exceed fine motor skills only in males with Down syndrome. Though heart disease has a significant effect on gross and fine motor performance, cognitive performance is consistently higher than motor performance, even in the presence of heart disease.

Hand strength is not a predictor of hand dominance. Grasp and other hand function is below the norm for non-Down syndrome children, but shows a wide variability in grip strength.

References

Ager, C., Olivett, B., & Johnson, C. (1984). Grasp and pinch strength in children five to twelve years old. *American Journal of Occupational Therapy, 38*, 107–113.

Carr, J. (1975). *Young children with Down syndrome*, (pp. 20–39). London: Butterworths.

Erhardt, R.P. (1982). Developmental hand dysfunction. *Evolution of the assessment*, (pp. 49–67). Laurel, MD.: Ramsco Publishers.

Harris, S.R. (1981). Relationship of mental and motor development in Down syndrome infants. *Physical and Occupational Therapy in Pediatrics, 1*, 13–18.

Harris, S.R. (1983). Comparative performance levels of female and male infants with Down syndrome. *Physical and Occupational Therapy in Pediatrics, 3*, 15–21.

Harris, S.R. (1984). Down syndrome. In S.K. Campbell, *Paediatric Neurologic Physical Therapy*, (pp. 169–204). New York: Churchill Living Stone.

LaVeck, B., & LaVeck, G.D. (1977). Sex differences in development among young children with Down syndrome. *Journal of Pediatrics, 91*(5), 767–769.

Mathiowetz, V., Weimer, D.M., & Federman, S.M. (1986). Grip and pinch strengths norms for 6–19 year olds. *American Journal of Occupational Therapy, 40* (10), 705–711.

Morris, A.F., Vaughan, S.E., & Vaccano, P. (1982). Measurements of neuromuscular tone and strength in Down's syndrome children. *Journal of Mental Deficiency Research, 26* (1), 41–46.

Schnell, R. (1984). *Psychomotor development. The young child with Down syndrome.* S.M. Pueschel Ed., pp. 207–226. New York: Human Sciences Press Inc.

Zausmer, E., & Shea, A. (1984). Motor development. The young child with Down syndrome. S.M. Pueschel (Ed.), (pp. 143–204). New York: The Human Sciences Press, Inc.

8
Problems in Feeding

DON C. VAN DYKE, LINDA LUSARDI PETERSON, AND MARTY NOVAK HOFFMAN

Introduction

A review of a feeding history questionnaire given to 190 parents with children with Down syndrome reveals that 49% answered affirmatively to the question, "were feeding problems present?" Studies of feeding patterns have supported the idea that normal motor development follows a systematic time table (Alexander, 1980). In children with Down syndrome, the sequence may be delayed. Abnormal feeding patterns and/or motor dysfunction have been identified in children with specific clinical neurologic presentations such as cerebral palsy (Blockley & Miller, 1971; Morris, 1977). Recently, clinical studies of severe feeding dysfunction have been reported in genetic/teratogenic syndromes (Van Dyke et al., 1982).

Multiple cranial skeletal differences in the child with Down syndrome may have a significant influence on feeding skills. The palate in a child with this syndrome is often short and narrow. This underdevelopment of the maxilla may alter the position of the muscles used for chewing. The tongue in some individuals is normal in size, but in others it may be large or appear large due to the existence of a small oral cavity secondary to midfacial hypoplasia (Hunt, 1981; Gisel, Lange, Niman, 1984; Smith, 1982). Many children with Down syndrome are mouthbreathers, due to a small oral cavity, enlargement of the tonsils, and/or decreased nasal passages. Generalized facial/oral hypotonia also contributes to poor lip closure, poor suck, poor tongue control, and difficulties with jaw stability. All of these factors may result in delays in oral motor skills (Gisel, et al., 1984; Hunt, 1982).

Oral motor patterns involve complex organized movements of the jaws, lips, cheeks, palate, and tongue. Jaw movements are crucial to the efficacy of chewing. It has been noted that children with Down syndrome demonstrate a reluctance to chew food and a preference to suck on items until swallowed. Gisel et al. (1984) studied the chewing movements of 26 children with Down syndrome, ages 4 to 5 years, and concluded that these children chew at a rate comparable to normal children, but that the duration of the chewing was prolonged per bite of food. This may reflect their reluctance or inability to chew food vigorously. These children also tended to hold food in their mouths for brief periods without chewing, and demonstrated difficulty in moving food from side to side wth their tongues.

In a study by Calvert et al. (1970), parents of 40 children with Down syndrome, ages 1 to 12 years, were interviewed regarding feeding problems. Specific eating problems identified in these children were: (1) difficulty using eating utensils; (2) trouble eating meat or chewing food; and (3) difficulty sucking, regurgitating and drinking from a cup. In the older child with chewing problems, liquids or food with soft textures were often substituted.

A chart review of 49 children with Down syndrome, ages 6 months to 6 years, found that 80% of the children studied had problems related to food or feeding (Pipes & Holm, 1980). Twenty-seven percent of the children refused anything but strained food, even when they were developmentally ready. This problem was particularly evident in the children between 25 and 36 months of age. A nutritional and feeding intervention program was established, and in 21 of these children, most nutritional, behavioral, and developmental problems surrounding foods were eliminated.

A longitudinal study by Cullen, Cronk, Pueschel, Schnell, and Reed (1981) evaluated the social and developmental feeding skills of 89 children with Down syndrome. Of the 89 children studied, 17 who had moderate or severe heart defects were more delayed in chewing, feeding and independent spoon use than those with mild heart defects. Overall, the feeding milestones of these children followed the same developmental sequence as that of non retarded children, but at a slower rate. Feeding milestones in the children ages 12 to 18 months were delayed in only 10%. After 18 months, they were delayed 20–30%. Females with Down syndrome reach feeding milestones earlier; usually less than two months before the males, which is not statistically significant.

Methods and Patient Population

Of 190 individuals with Down syndrome, feeding histories were obtained on 184. A review of these feeding histories showed that, by parental report, 49% had feeding problems. However, over an extended period of time, caregivers reported that only 31% of these individuals reported significant feeding problems.

Over an 18-month period of time, a subgroup of 58 of the 190 children with Down syndrome were studied regarding oral motor development in feeding. The oral motor screening form was developed to assess oral control, muscle tone, and reflexes (see Table 8.1). The subgroup consisted of 58 children ages 0.1 to 19 years, most of whom were less than 3 years of age. When possible, parents were requested to bring food to the evaluation in order to observe feeding skills. A majority of the information was obtained from questioning the parents. Additional areas assessed included breathing patterns, drooling,

TABLE 8.1. Oral motor assessment.[a]

	Present	Absent	Comments
Oral reflexes			
Rooting			
Gag			
Bite			
Suck swallow			
Tactile response			Intraoral/extraoral
	Normal	Abnormal	Comments
Facial tone			Cheeks/lips
Oral control			
Swallowing			Mouth open/mouth closed
Breathing			Mouth/nose/both
Drooling			While eating only/ mild/moderate/severe/teething
Sucking			
Swallowing (Liquids)			
Swallowing (Solids)			
Chewing			Occlusion/mouth open or closed. vertical/horizontal/rotary
Lip closure			Open at will/around cup/straw/spoon
Tongue Control			Directional movement/ protruding/thrusting/ eating interference

[a]*Source:* Linda Lusardi Peterson, 1984.

sucking, swallowing of liquids and solids, chewing ability, lip closure, and tongue control. A developmental feeding table modified from Gessell and Ilg was used as a reference for feeding skills (Pipes & Holm, 1980). This table relates feeding to developmental levels rather than chronological age, and lists skills that can be used as guidelines to assess feeding readiness. This tool was also given to parents as a guideline, to encourage them to try something new, or to confirm the efficacy of their present feeding intervention program.

Results

A review of feeding histories in the newborn showed 57% of the mothers of children with Down syndrome breastfed their children at some time. A large percentage of mothers (43%) never breastfed; 81% bottle-fed at some time in the child's first year of life, with only 19% never bottle-feeding (See Table 8.2). The significance of this number is that a smaller number of mothers with infants with Down syndrome breastfeed than other mothers, while a greater number of these mothers use both breast and bottle to feed their child during his or her first year of life.

This study found slight hypotonia of the oral region to be a common finding in children with Down syndrome, with 41% having some degree of oral hypotonia. The most common concerns noted were difficulties in chewing,

TABLE 8.2. Feeding history in Down syndrome.

Problems	N	Yes (%)	No (%)
Feeding problems (newborn nursery)	177	87 (49)	90 (50)
Feeding problems in general (0.1–19 yrs)	179	55 (31)	124 (69)
Breast feed (at any time)	184	105 (57)	79 (43)
Bottle feed (at any time)	171	139 (81)	32 (19)
Feeds self independently	178	106 (60)	72 (40)

TABLE 8.3. Feeding problems by age in 58 Down syndrome individuals.

Age (years)	Non-Interfering tongue thrust	Interfering tongue thrust	Chewing difficulty	Poor lip closure	Choking/ gagging	Total problems by age
<1	7	6	—	2	2	17
1	7	3	4	2	2	18
2	5	3	3	—	1	12
3	1	—	5	1	—	7
4	3	1	2	—	1	7
5	—	1	3	5	—	9
6	1	1	—	—	2	4
7	1	1	2	—	—	4
8	2	—	—	—	—	2
9	2	—	2	—	2	6
10	—	—	1	—	—	1
11	1	—	2	—	—	3
12	1	—	—	—	—	1
13	—	—	1	—	—	1
14	2	—	—	—	—	2
15	2	—	—	—	1	3
16–19	—	—	—	—	—	—
Total	35	16	25	10	11	97[a]
%	60	28	43	17	19	N/A

[a]Number of problems is greater than 58 since some children had multiple feeding problems.

poor lip closure, and choking and gagging on food. Also noted was a tongue thrust, not severe enough to interfere with feeding, which was most commonly seen in the children younger than 3 years. Only 28% were noted to have a tongue thrust severe enough to interfere with feeding. Other problem areas noted were difficulty in chewing (43%), poor lip closure (17%), and choking and gagging (19%). Many children had feeding problems in multiple areas (see Table 8.3).

Discussion

In individuals with Down syndrome, eating problems are common but usually minor in nature. In a survey of parents, it would appear that 60% are totally independent in feeding by early childhood. The most common oral problems are slight oral hypotonia, tongue thrust, difficulties in chewing, poor lip closure, and choking and gagging on food. Feeding programs to help parents and children to deal with these problems are important and should continue to be included in developmental programs. The success of existing programs may in fact be partly responsible for the large number of persons with Down syndrome who are becoming independent in feeding, regardless of minor (though present) feeding problems.

Summary

Fewer numbers of mothers of infants with Down syndrome breastfed than did mothers of non-Down syndrome infants. The frequent presence of hypotonia in the oral region may explain why bottle feeding/breast feeding is more popular. Common feeding concerns of parents of Down syndrome infants were difficulties in chewing, lip closing, and choking/gagging. Although some children had multiple feeding problems, they were usually of a minor nature. Most Down syndrome children were totally independent in feeding by early childhood.

References

Alexander, R. (1980). *Early Feeding, Sound Production and Prelinguistic Cognitive Development in Their Relationship to Gross Motor Development.* Madison, WI: Curative Rehabilitation Center.

Blockley, J., & Miller, G. (1971). Feeding techniques with cerebral palsied children. *Physiotherapy, 57* (7), 300–308.

Calvert, S.D., Vivian, V.M., & Calvert, G.P. (1970). Dietary adequacy, feeding practices, and eating behavior of children with Down syndrome. *Journal of American Dietetic Association, 69*, 152–156.

Cullen, S.M., Cronk, G.E., Pueschel, S.M., Schnell, R.R., & Reed, R.B. (1981). Social development and feeding milestones of young Down Syndrome children. *American Journal of Mental Deficiency, 85* (4), 410–415.

Gisel, E.G., Lange, L.J., & Niman, C.W. (1984). Chewing cycles in four- and five-year old Down syndrome children: A comparison of eating efficacy with normal children. *Journal of Occupational Therapy, 38* (10), 666–670.

Hunt, P.J. (1982). *Oral Motor Dysfunction in Down Syndrome: Contributing Factors and Interventions.* New York: Haworth Press.

Morris, S.E. (1977). *Program Guidelines for Children with Feeding Problems.* Edison, NJ: Childcraft Educational Corp., 48.

Pipes, P.L., & Holm, V.A. (1980). Feeding children with Down's syndrome. *Journal of American Dietetic Association, 77* (5), 277–282.

Smith, D.W. (1982). *Recognizable Patterns of Human Malformations.* Philadelphia: W.B. Saunders.

Van Dyke, D.C., Mackay, L., & Zlaylek, E.N. (1982). Management of severe feeding dysfunction in children with fetal alcohol syndrome. *Clinical Pediatrics, 21* (6), 336–339.

9
Nutrition Assessment of the Child with Down Syndrome

MARION TAYLOR BAER, JAN WALDRON, HEATHER GUMM, DON C. VAN DYKE, AND HYEJUNG CHANG

Introduction

Nutrition assessment of children is based upon careful evaluation of several parameters that, taken together, provide an indication of their nutritional health. These parameters include clinical (physical examination, anthropometry), dietary (present nutrient intake, historical data), and biochemical (nutrient stores, functional tests) measures. Often, children with special needs also require an assessment of feeding skills, as their delayed or abnormal development may affect food intake. Of these measures, anthropometry, or the measurement of growth and body composition in the child, is the most objective indicator of that child's nutritional status. Decreased nutrient intake, due to feeding problems or poor diet, will ultimately be reflected in poor growth and/or decreased fat and muscle mass. Overnutrition, due to overeating and/or decreased physical activity, ultimately is reflected in increased fat stores.

Nutrition assessment of the child with Down syndrome is complicated by a number of problems that affect either the nutritional status of the child or its assessment. The purpose of this chapter is to outline some of these problems, to present some preliminary results of the nutrition component of this cross-sectional study, and to provide some recommendations regarding nutrition assessment of the child with Down syndrome.

Problems in Nutrition Assessment of the Child with Down Syndrome

Growth Problems

Anthropometric assessment of the child with Down syndrome is complicated by the fact that the disorder has been associated with a number of abnormalities related to growth, including short stature, decreased head circumference, and altered growth patterns.

Several studies reviewed by Cronk indicate that while lengths/heights in the Down syndrome population are significantly lower than the norm, the period in which most significant growth failure occurs is during the first five years of life (Cronk, 1978; Cronk et al., 1988). This is also true of black children with Down syndrome (Ershow, 1986). The importance of growth during early childhood was corroborated by a longitudinal study by Rarick and Seefeldt (1974). Their study showed that although prepubertal children with Down syndrome were shorter as a group than normal children, their *growth velocity* between 7 and 18 years of age was not significantly different from that of normal children during the same growth period. Evaluations of sitting heights in the population with Down syndrome indicated that the short stature may be due to decreased leg length (Jaswal & Jaswal, 1981; Rarick & Seefeldt, 1974).

Head circumferences, compared to the National Center for Health Statistics (NCHS) reference data, indicate that children with Down syndrome are significantly microcephalic. However, Cronk and Pueschel (1984) noted that neither males nor females could be classified as truly microcephalic since head circumferences were never two standard deviations below the mean once stature was taken into account.

Congenital heart disease occurs in approximately 40% of children with Down syndrome (see Chapter 1). Particularly in cyanotic and general heart disease this may have a significant effect on nutritional needs and growth. Previous studies of growth in children with Down syndrome who had mild congenital heart disease did not indicate compromised growth. However, those individuals with moderate to severe heart disease experienced significant growth delays (Cronk et al., 1988; Cronk & Pueschel, 1984; Pueschel, 1984).

Feeding Problems

Feeding difficulties are common among children with Down syndrome (Calvert, et al., 1976; Palmer, 1978a). A retrospective chart review by Pipes and Holm (1980) of 49 children with Down syndrome from 6 months to 6½ years of age showed that 80% had one or more feeding problems. The delayed development of feeding skills in children with Down syndrome (see Chapter 8) may be the consequence of problems with sucking, swallowing, chewing, and self-feeding, which are commonly related to oral hypotonia, small midface and oral cavity leading to mouth breathing and tongue protrusion and delayed and abnormal dentition. It may also be related to inappropriate feeding practices on the part of caregivers who do not recognize when the child is developmentally ready to acquire a new skill (Pipes & Holm, 1980). Interdisciplinary longitudinal early intervention studies have indicated that feeding milestones in children with Down syndrome can be achieved earlier, with appropriate parental guidance (Cullen, et al., 1981; Pipes & Holm, 1980).

Although several of the documented reasons for the growth problems in Down syndrome such as congenital heart disease and feeding problems, are potentially nutrition related, it is still not clear what role nutrition plays in their etiology. A Japanese study of secular growth trends indicated that the increase in stature over time seen in normal infants in Japan was not seen in those with Down syndrome, suggesting that environmental causes of the short stature do not play a major role (Hoshi, 1979). It is also possible that the growth abnormalities and short stature seen in children with Down syndrome are related to other manifestations of the disorder such as thyroid dysfunction (Sharov, 1981) or other metabolic differences.

Obesity

Depending on the investigator's definition, mild to significant obesity has been reported in individuals with Down syndrome, beginning in 1955 (Benda & Mann, 1955; Chumlea & Cronk, 1981; Cronk, 1978, Pipes & Holm, 1980; Walker, 1955). The etiology of the "obesity" has not been thoroughly explained, however (Cronk & Chumlea, 1985), and other, more recent, studies have failed to confirm a high incidence in children reared at home (Calvert et al., 1976; Stedman & Eichorn, 1964), which suggests environmental, rather than disorder-related, causes. Culley and co-workers (1965) studied the energy intake of 23 institutionalized children with Down syndrome who were considered to be well-nourished. They found it to be comparable to that of noninstitutionalized children (Beal, 1961) when it was expressed as calories per centimeter of height (15.3 kcal/cm for normal males versus 16.3 kcal/cm for males with Down syndrome; 13.5 kcal/cm for normal females versus 14.3 kcal/cm for females with Down syndrome). Findings in that study suggest that the recommended dietary allowance (RDA) for *age* may overestimate the energy needs of the child with Down syndrome. In addition, the decreased activity level of these children, many of whom are hypotonic in infancy and have poor gross motor skills as they grow older, may further reduce energy needs.

Biochemical Abnormalities

Biochemical abnormalities suggestive of poor nutritional status have been reported with respect to certain nutrients. These include vitamins A, C, E, thiamin, niacin (Matin, 1981), pyridoxine and the mineral zinc. Of these, vitamin A, pyridoxine, and zinc have received the most attention.

Vitamin A

Vitamin A nutriture in persons with Down syndrome has been investigated because of the high incidence of hyperkeratosis and upper respiratory tract infections that have been observed in this population, as well as impaired dark adaptation (Griffith & Behrman, 1966). Serum vitamin A levels have been reported to be lower in individuals with Down syndrome (Appleton et al.,

1964; Palmer, 1978b; Sobel et al., 1958), possibly due to malabsorption (Auld et al., 1959; Palmer, 1978b). However, other workers have failed to confirm these findings (Barden, 1977; Cutress et al., 1976), or to associate low serum vitamin A levels with hyperkeratosis (Martin et al., 1981). Barden (1977), however, also noted very high carotene levels in his institutionalized subjects with and without Down syndrome as compared to normal subjects ($p < 0.001$), apparently due to the high content of carotene in the institutional diet. He postulated that the normal serum vitamin A levels he found may be a function of carotene "loading" since the carotene/vitamin A ratios were also significantly higher than controls ($p < 0.001$) and that there may be an inefficient mechanism for carotene-to–vitamin A conversion.

In an intervention study, Palmer (1978b) paired children with Down syndrome, who had low serum vitamin A levels, with their normal siblings and supplemented half the pairs with 1,000 i.u. vitamin A/month. At the end of the five-month trial, plasma vitamin A levels in the treated children with Down syndrome were no longer significantly lower than those of normal controls, although they were still lower than those of treated controls. Palmer also reported a significant decrease in the incidence of infection and a reduction in serum IgG only in those children with Down syndrome who were treated, leading her to hypothesize that the increased susceptibility to infection may be related to abnormalities in vitamin A metabolism.

ZINC

Low serum zinc has also been reported (Bjorksten et al., 1980; Gofman et al., 1962; Milunsky et al., 1970) in persons with Down syndrome. Because of the importance of zinc to immune function and because immune function appears to be compromised in this disorder (Costello & Webber, 1976; Khan et al., 1975; Levin, et al., 1975; Pueschel & Pezzullo, 1985), Bjorksten and coworkers (1980) postulated that zinc deficiency may partially explain the increased susceptibility to infection in Down syndrome. They were able to show that two months of zinc supplementation (135 mg elemental zinc per day) not only raised serum zinc to normal levels but improved several measures of abnormal immune function in 12 children with Down syndrome. It is not known, however, whether dietary inadequacies were the cause of the apparent zinc deficiency, or if persons with Down syndrome have increased needs or turnover/excretion of this nutrient. Nor has the known interrelationship between zinc and vitamin A been investigated in Down syndrome. Since both of these nutrients are essential for normal growth, these questions need to be explored.

PYRIDOXINE

Children with Down syndrome have also been reported to have abnormalities in pyridoxine (vitamin B-6) and/or tryptophan metabolism, as well as abnormally low levels of blood serotonin (Tu & Zellweger, 1965). These observations have led some clinicians, concerned about the decreased muscle tone common to children with Down syndrome, to attempt to treat this symptom with 5-hydroxytryptophan, the immediate precursor of serotonin, or pyridoxine, the vitamin cofactor necessary for the reaction. The results of such trials have been mixed, but have generally been negative (Baselon et al., 1976; Partington et al., 1971; Pueschel, 1984; Weise et al., 1974). Again, the studies did not adequately address the question of the overall vitamin B-6 status of these children, reporting no dietary information, for example.

The possibility, perhaps legitimate, that the need for certain nutrients may be increased because of the presence of extra chromosomal material, has led some to suggest that dietary supplementation with magadoses of several vitamins and minerals can help to "normalize" children with Down syndrome (Harrel et al., 1981; Turkel, 1975) (see Chapter 19). However, studies carefully designed to test this hypothesis have not yielded positive results (Bennetts et al., 1983; Smith et al., 1984; Weathers, 1983).

Present Study

Purpose

Although short stature and slow growth rate have been clearly associated with malnutrition in other population groups, no study has yet been undertaken to determine the potential role of poor nutrition in the etiology of poor growth in children with Down syndrome. Similarly, although the prevalence of obesity appears to be greater among children with Down syndrome, its relationship to dietary intake has not been documented. Nor has the "obesity" been investigated using techniques to analyze body composition in order to determine whether the excessive weight is indeed due to excessive fat and not to other possible causes such as large frame size relative to stature or greater relative trunk length in proportion to stature (Cronk & Chumlea, 1985).

The purpose of this cross-sectional study was to carefully document dietary intake as well as growth parameters in a large group of children with Down syndrome and to relate these to information regarding their early and present feeding histories as well as their cardiac and thyroid status. In addition, measurement of skinfolds was made to further define body composition in an attempt to determine the prevalance of true obesity in our population. The dietary and most of the anthropometric data have not yet been fully analyzed and will be published elsewhere. No biochemical determinations were performed. The following is a report of the preliminary, largely descriptive analysis of the anthropometric data only.

Subjects

The patient population, described in detail in the Introduction and Appendix 1, consisted of 190 individuals with Down syndrome. All types of Down syndrome (i.e., Trisomy 21, translocation, mosaic) were included. Of the 190, 77 (41%) had suspected heart disease; 14 were determined to have only innocent murmurs, leaving 63 (33%) with documented heart disease ranging from mild to very severe (Chapter 4).

Dietary and anthropometric data were collected for the 187 individuals who were 18 years old and younger; 97 girls and 90 boys. Thirteen of these children were judged by clinicians (pediatrics/pediatric cardiology), based on chart review, parental report, and examination, to have heart disease severe enough to have a probable ($N = 5$) or definite ($N = 8$) effect on growth parameters. These problems, as well as the age and sex of the children, appear in Table 9.1.

Methods

The nutrition evaluation was conducted in two parts. The first part consisted of a nutrition history questionnaire and a three-day food record; the second was anthropometry.

TABLE 9.1. Cardiac defects judged by clinicians to affect growth.

Probable effect on growth (Moderate heart disease)			
Pt. #	Sex	Age	Defect
71	F	4 mo.	AV canal
14	F	12 mo.	VSD
40	F	16.5 mo.	ASD/VSD
32	F	36 mo.	ASD/VSD
171	F	5 yrs.	Endocardial cushion defect/polycythemia
Definite effect on growth (Severe heart disease)			
Pt. #	Sex	Age	Defect
123	F	19 mo.	Absent mitral valve
			VSD
			Aortic stenosis
			VSD/ASD
			Pulmonary ductus arteriosis
89	M	21 mo.	Tetrology of fallot
18	M	21 mo.	Mitral valve regurgitation in AV canal
167	M	30 mo.	Pulmonary hypertension
			Partial anomalous pulmonary vitus return
137	F	30 mo.	Mitral valve regurgitation in AV canal
71	F	5 yr., 2 mo.	ASD/VSD
			Pulmonary ductus arteriosus
			Mitral insufficiency
29	F	6 yrs.	AV canal
			Pulmonary ductus arteriosus
			Mitral valve regurgitation (post repair)
			Tricuspid valve regurgitation
105	F	10 yrs., 7 mo.	Mitral valve prolapse
			AV canal
			Pulmonary hypertension

The nutrition history questionnaire and a three-day food record were completed by the family prior to the child being evaluated. During the interview session a dietitian reviewed and clarified the questionnaire and food records with the primary care provider. Food models and common measuring devices were used to help determine quantities. A commercially available computerized data base, the "Food Processor" (Geltz & Geltz, 1984), was used to analyse the food records. These analyses are not yet complete.

The anthropometry was performed on each individual by two nutritionists trained in the use of standardized anthropometric techniques (see Appendix 10.1). Specific measurements taken were: recumbent and crown-rump lengths on children 36 months or less; standing and sitting heights in children older than 36 months; weight; head circumference; midarm circumference (MAC); triceps skinfold (TSF); and subscapular skinfold (SSF). Arm-muscle circumference (AMC) was derived mathematically. All measurements were compared to reference data according to chronological age and sex. A list of reference data used for specific measurements appears as Table 9.2.

Preliminary Results and Discussion

Effect of Cardiac Status on Growth Parameters

Analysis of variance indicated that the effect of the child's cardiac status was significant ($p < 0.05$) only for weight and length/height as compared to NCHS reference data, and length/height as compared to Down syndrome–specific data (Cronk et al., 1988) when the entire sample was considered. The majority of the children (174/187) had no heart disease or mild heart disease only; there were no differences seen between these groups. The differences were signifi-

TABLE 9.2. Reference data for comparison of growth measurements.

Anthropometric parameters	Reference data
Height/age Weight/age Weight/length or height	NCHS growth charts— Birth to 36 months, and 2 to 18 years of age Frisancho (1981).
Head circumference	NCHS birth to 36 months Nellhaus (1968) > 36 months
Triceps skin fold (TSF) Midarm circumference (MAC) Arm muscle circumference (AMC)	Frisancho (1981) 1–18 years Frisancho (1974) < 1 year
Subscapular skinfold (SSF)	Fomon (1977) < 1 year; Johnson, C.L., Fulwood, R., Abraham, S. et al. (1981) > 1 year
Children with Down syndrome	Cronk et al. (1988)

TABLE 9.3. Comparison of growth parameters in children with Down syndrome with or without cardiac problems.

Growth parameter	Normal distribution	NoCHD/ mean(N)	CHD/ mean(N)	P-value
Male				
Length (cm)	No	101.15 (62)	89.90 (26)	0.1168 (w)
Weight (kg)	No	21.53 (62)	15.85 (26)	0.0864 (w)
Head circumference (cm)	Yes	47.10 (61)	44.78 (26)	0.0140 (t)[a]
Crown-rump Length (cm)	Yes	47.55 (27)	45.79 (14)	0.3279 (t)
Mid-arm circumference (cm)	No	18.73 (62)	16.73 (24)	0.0274 (w)[a]
Subscapular skin-fold (mm)	No	9.03 (62)	7.92 (25)	0.3675 (w)
Triceps skin-fold (mm)	No	10.96 (62)	9.54 (24)	0.2536 (w)
Arm-muscle circumference (cm)	No	15.32 (62)	13.73 (24)	0.0611 (w)
Female				
Length (cm)	No	92.94 (61)	87.15 (36)	0.5015 (w)
Weight (kg)	No	18.88 (61)	14.21 (36)	0.3242 (w)
Head circumference (cm)	Yes	45.04 (60)	44.29 (36)	0.3290 (t)
Crown-rump (cm)	No	46.08 (29)	45.28 (18)	0.9302 (w)
Mid-arm circumference (cm)	No	18.48 (60)	16.75 (35)	0.1534 (w)'
Subscapular skin-fold (mm)	No	10.56 (59)	7.92 (35)	0.1497 (w)
Triceps skin-fold (mm)	No	12.26 (60)	9.63 (35)	0.0289 (w)[a]
Arm-muscle circumference (cm)	No	14.77 (60)	13.67 (35)	0.1857 (w)

(t) = *t*-test (parameteric method);
(w) = Wilcoxon Rank Sum Test (nonparametric method)
[a]Significant at 0.05 level

cant only between those with no or mild cardiac problems, and those judged to have severe cardiac problems. This confirms the findings of others (Cronk et al., 1988; Cronk & Pueschel, 1984; Pueschel, 1984).

All of the children with cardiac disease were grouped (CHD) and compared to those free of it (no CHD). For each anthropometric variable we checked the normality of the distribution of the measured values (mean differences). If the distribution was normal, the *p*-value was calculated using a parametric test (matched *t*-test). If normality was not demonstrated, the *p*-value was calculated using a nonparametric method (Wilcoxon Rank Sum test). Although all means were lower in the CHD group, few significant differences were seen (Table 9.3), and there were none in length/height or weight parameters. The reason is probably the small number of children with moderate or severe problems (13/187) included in the sample. Because there were few differences and because we wish to compare our data to those of Cronk and her coworkers, we chose to include the CHD children in our subsequent analyses.

For the purposes of this chapter we will concentrate on the preliminary authropometic analyses of the largest group of children—those 48 months and younger. These data are purely descriptive—no statistical analyses have yet been performed. We look here only at the percentages of the children, aged 0–24 months and 25–48 months, who appear to be at increased risk for under- or overnutrition as compared to available reference data.

Risk Indicators for Undernutrition (see Table 9.4)

Prevalence of Short Stature

Length or height below the 5th percentile for age, using the NCHS reference data, is commonly considered to indicate short stature in the normal population. In the total study group, 58% of males and 62% of females fell below the 5th percentile. For children less than 48 months, the percentages were similar (59% and 63%), confirming the findings of others that the growth retardation occurs early in life (Cronk et al., 1988). However, when the data are compared to the Down syndrome–specific data (Cronk et al., 1988), the prevalence of short stature in children less than 48 months approaches the expected 5% (10% of males, no females). Similarly, 9% of the children under 48 months fell below the 10th percentile using Cronk's reference data. Further statistical analyses will be done to determine how well our data fit with those of Cronk and her colleagues.

Prevalence of Microcephaly

Consistent with the findings of others, 71% of females and 84% of males under four show microcephaly, defined as head circumference below the 5th percentile, compared to normal children. It appears to be more pronounced in the older subgroup (2–4 years) where 95% fall below the 5th percentile (Nellhaus, 1968).

Prevalence of Underweight

Weight for age below the 5th percentile, using appropriate reference data, puts a child at risk for being underweight and needs to be explored before the child's growth is compromised. Some clinicians are concerned if weight for age is below the 10th percentile. However, many children with Down syndrome fall into this range and may show no other indicators of undernutrition when their measurements are compared to NCHS reference data. In our population, weight of 32% of the children fell below the 5th percentile, and nearly half were below the 10th percentile. However, using the Down syndrome–specific reference data, it can be seen that those percentages change to 3% and 7%, respectively. This is within the rnage of the expected prevalence.

Weight for height, which is an age-independent parameter, can also be used as a measure of underweight. The number of children under 48 months who were at risk using this criterion was 14% (below the 10th percentile) and 5% (below the 5th percentile); again, this is within the expected range. However, there appears to be a sex difference here, with more males at possible risk.

TABLE 9.4. Children with Down syndrome under 48 months at risk for undernutrition

		0–24 Months					25–48 Months					0–48 Months		
Criterion	Percentile	Males n = 30–31	%	Females n = 39	%	Total %	Males n = 17–19	%	Females n = 19–20	%	Total %	Males %	Females %	Total %
Length or height (NCHS)	<10	20/30	67	27/39	69	68	17/19	89	18/20	90	90	73	76	75
	<5	15/30	50	19/39	49	49	14/19	68	18/20	90	82	59	63	61
(Cronk et al., 1988)	<10	2/30	7	2/39	5	6	5/19	26	2/20	11	18	12	7	9
	<5	1/30	3	0/39	0	1	4/19	21	0/20	0	10	10	0	5
Weight (NCHS)	<10	16/30	53	15/39	38	45	13/19	68	9/20	47	56	59	41	49
	<5	10/30	33	8/39	21	26	11/19	58	6/20	32	44	43	24	32
(Cronk et al., 1988)	<10	1/30	3	0/39	0	1	4/19	21	3/20	16	18	10	5	7
	<5	0/30	0	0/39	0	0	3/19	16	0/20	0	8	6	0	3
Weight for length/height (NCHS)	<10	6/30	20	3/39	8	13	5/19	26	1/20	5	15	22	7	14
	<5	2/30	7	1/39	2.5	4	2/19	10.5	0/20	0	5	8	2	5
Midarm circumference (Frisancho 1974, 1981)	<10	6/31	19	4/39	10	14	2/17	12	1/19	5.5	8	17	9	12
	<5	3/31	10	1/39	2.5	6	1/17	6	1/19	5	5.5	8	2	6

Arm muscle circumference														
(Frisancho	<10	0/31	0	1/39	2.5	1	0/17	0	0/19	0	0	0	2	<1
1974, 1981)	<5	0/31	0	1/39	2.5	1	0/17	0	0/19	0	0	0	2	<1
Skin fold thickness														
Triceps														
(Frisancho	<10	1/31	3	3/39	8	6	1/17	6	1/19	5	5.5	4	7	6
1974, 1981)	<5	1/31	3	1/39	2.5	3	1/17	6	1/19	5	5.5	4	3	4
Subscapular														
(Fomon)	<10	6/31	19	11/39	28	24	1/18	5.5	1/19	5	5.5	14	21	18
	<5	0/31	0	0/39	0	0	0/18	0	0/19	0	0	0	0	0
(NCHS	<10						1/18	5.5	1/19	5	6.5			
Johnson)	<5						0/18	0	0/19	0	0			
Head circumference														
(NCHS,	<10	24/31	77	30/39	77	77	18/19	95	20/20	100	98	84	85	84
Nellhaus)	<5	24/31	77	23/39	59	67	18/19	95	19/20	95	95	84	71	77

Indication of Wasting

Skinfold Measurements (Fat Stores)

Measurement of weight alone is not always a good estimate of the amount of body fat, since weight also represents bone and muscle and these vary from child to child. The amount of body fat can be estimated indirectly by measuring "skinfolds," which include the layer of fat under the skin, on the back of the upper arm (triceps) and below the scapula (subscapular).

Triceps skinfold measurements in the children under 48 months indicate that 4% of the population fell below the 5th percentile; 6% fell below the 10th percentile. There were no subscapular skinfolds below the 5th percentile. This suggests no increased prevalence of low fat stores in these children. However, 18% of those under 48 months did fall below the 10th percentile for subscapular skinfold measurements when the data are compared to those of Fomon (1977; the only reference data that include infants 0–12 months). Furthermore, it can be seen in Table 9.4 that most of those children were in the 0- to 24-month age range. This may or may not indicate increased risk, since the Fomon data represent a limited population of normal children.

Midarm and Arm-Muscle Circumferences (Somatic Protein Stores)

Midarm circumference, in conjunction with skinfold measurements, can be used to estimate muscle mass, or somatic protein stores. In the under-48-month subgroup, 6% of the children (8% males, 2% females) fell below the 5th percentile for midarm circumference, the expected prevalence. However, arm-muscle circumference measurements were higher; less than 1% of the total group had values below the 5th percentile (no males, 2% of females). This suggests that our population of children with Down syndrome had no undernutrition severe enough to cause muscle wasting.

Risk Indicators for Overnutrition (see Table 9.5)

Prevalence of Overweight

Because of the high incidence of short stature, it is not appropriate to use only the NCHS reference data for weight to evaluate children with Down syndrome. In fact, only 2% of the children under four years fell into the high-risk category (> 95th percentile) for normal children, whereas 6% could be considered to be overweight if the Down syndrome–specific reference data are used (Table 9.5). Again, this is close to the expected prevalence and close to the percentage of our sample under four years (5.5%), which can be considered to be at risk for obesity based on NCHS reference data for weight for stature.

There appears to be an increased risk for overweight based on weight for stature in the 25- to 48-month-olds (10% above the 95th percentile). And, when all of the subjects 18 years and under are considered, the number whose weight for height is greater than the 95th percentile (NCHS) jumps to 18% for

TABLE 9.5. Children with Down syndrome under 48 months at risk for obesity.

Criterion	Percentile	0–24 Months Males n = 30–32	%	Females n = 39	%	Total %	25–48 Months Males n = 17–19	%	Females n = 19–20	%	Total %	0–48 Months Males %	Females %	Total %
Weight														
(NCHS)	>90	2/30	7	1/39	2.5	4	1/19	5	0/20	0	2.5	6	2	4
	>95	1/30	3	1/39	2.5	3	0/19	0	0/20	0	0	2	2	2
(Cronk et al., 1988)	>90	4/30	13	3/39	8	10	1/19	5	0/20	0	2.5	10	5	7
	>95	4/30	13	2/39	5	9	1/19	5	0/20	0	2.5	10	3	6
Weight for length/ height (NCHS)	>90	4/30	13	2/39	5	9	2/19	10.5	6/20	30	20.5	12	14	13
	>95	1/30	3	1/39	2.5	3	1/19	5	3/20	15	10	4	7	5.5
Skin fold thickness														
Triceps														
(NCHS, Frisancho 1974, 1981)	>90	3/31	10	1/39	2.5	6	0/17	0	1/19	5	3	6	3	5
	>95	1/31	3	0/39	0	1	0/17	0	0/19	0	0	2	0	<1
Subscapular														
(Fomon)	>90	4/31	13	3/39	8	10	6/18	33	6/19	32	32	20	16	18
	>95	0/31	0	0/39	0	0	1/18	5.5	0/19	0	3	2	0	<1
(NCHS Johnson 1981)	>90						3/18	17	8/19	42	30			
	>95						2/18	11	6/19	32	22			
Midarm circumference														
(Frisancho 1974, 1981)	>90	2/31	6	3/39	8	7	1/17	6	3/19	16	11	6	10	8
	>95	1/31	3	3/39	8	6	0/17	0	1/19	5	3	2	7	5
Arm muscle circumference														
(Frisancho 1974, 1981)	>90	1/31	3	5/39	13	8.5	2/17	12	4/19	21	17	6	16	11
	>95	1/31	3	5/39	13	8.5	2/17	12	4/19	21	17	6	16	11

males and 14% for females. This suggests a tendency to put on weight with age, and/or that preventive strategies associated with the increased emphasis on early intervention have been successful in helping caregivers to avoid inappropriate weight gain in the younger children (Cronk & Pueschel, 1984).

Skinfold Measurement

If triceps skinfold measurements are used as a criterion of obesity, the children with Down syndrome under four years also do not appear to be excessively overfat. Only 2% had triceps skinfolds greater than the 95th percentile (NCHS), which is, if anything, less than the expected prevalence. Subscapular skinfold, measurements also indicate that very few (2% of males, no females) of these children were at risk for obesity using the Fomon reference data. However, the subscapular skinfolds in this subgroup of children also indicate that 18%, about twice the expected prevalence, had measurements above the 90th percentile. The bulk of the high measurements was found in the 2- to 4-year-olds. Also when NCHS data are used to evaluate the skinfolds of the 2- to 4-year-olds, the prevalence jumps to 22% (11% males, 32% females) with measurements greater than the 95th percentile. This suggests that children with Down syndrome may have a different distribution of body fat, more truncal than peripheral. Also, although this was a cross-sectional study, the fact that this pattern appears in the 24- to 48-month-olds may indicate that the tendency to put on truncal weight develops after infancy. Analyses to determine other correlates (triceps, weight, weight for height, ponderal index) have not yet been completed.

Arm and Arm-Muscle Circumferences

The arm and arm-muscle circumferences suggest an important contribution of muscle mass to body weight in children with Down syndrome. Our preliminary analyses show that the midarm circumferences appear to fall in approximately the same ranges as those of normal children. Given the fact that children with Down syndrome are, as a group, considerably shorter and have shortened limbs (Jaswal & Jaswal, 1981), arms of normal circumference may give these children a stocky appearance. Furthermore, the normal arm circumferences are apparently due mainly to increased muscle mass. Not only are there few triceps skinfold measurements above the 90th percentile, but fewer than 1% of the children have an arm-muscle circumference less than even the 10th percentile, while 11% have arm-muscle circumferences above the 95th percentile. Furthermore, 79% of the boys and 65% of the girls in the 24- to 48-month age range have measurements above the 50th percentile (Johnson et al., 1981).

Recommendations for Nutrition Assessment of the Child with Down Syndrome

Nutrition assessment should be included as part of the overall interdisciplinary evaluation of the child with Down syndrome. Because most of the potential nutrition-related problems such as feeding difficulties, delayed milestones in the development of feeding skills, inappropriate food intake or inappropriate weight gain are preventable, anticipatory guidance and early intervention are especially important. Detailed recommendations for nutrition assessment and intervention for the child with Down syndrome can be found elsewhere (Palmer, 1978a; Pipes & Holm, 1980). A brief summary of the important factors to consider in assessment is included here as Appendix 10.2.

Summary

Based on preliminary, descriptive analyses of our growth data there appears to be little evidence of malnutrition serious enough to cause stunting in the children under 48 months of age in our sample. The short stature, slow growth rate, and microcephaly compared to normal reference data, which have been reported previously, were also seen in this subgroup. However, compared to Down syndrome–specific data, there was no more than the expected prevalence of short stature. Nor was there evidence of wasting, based either on arm circumference, arm-muscle circumference, or triceps skinfold measurements. There was a large number of children (24%) in the 0- to 24-month age range with subscapular skinfolds below the 10th percentile. However, the significance of this finding is not clear, especially since none fell below the 5th percentile.

Similarly, we saw little evidence of the expected high prevalence of overweight or obesity. Again, only the subscapular measurement indicated a greater than expected number of children at risk. In this case, the 25- to 48-month-olds appear to be at highest risk. The possibility that the data suggest a pattern of increased truncal fat deposition in children with Down syndrome needs to be explored, as does the apparent increased muscle mass based on a greater than expected number of large arm-muscle circumference measurements, again, especially in the 25- to 48-month-olds.

Further analyses will be undertaken to determine the significance of these findings, as well as those for the children in the sample over four years of age. The growth parameters will also be examined in light of the dietary data that remain to be analyzed and information related to development of feeding skills in these children.

Acknowledgement. The authors wish to thank Dr. Christine E. Cronk for her contributions to the preparation of this chapter.

References

Appleton, M.D., Haab, W., Carey, P.J., Castellino, F.J., Sehon, J.M., & Miraglia, R.J. (1964). Role of vitamin A in gammaglobulin biosynthesis and uric acid metabolism of mongoloids. *American Journal of Mental Deficiency, 69*, 324.

Auld, R.M., Pommer, A.M., Houch, J.C., & Burke, F.G. (1959). Vitamin A absorption in mongoloid children: a preliminary report. *American Journal of Mental Deficiency, 63*, 1010.

Barden, H.S. (1977). Vitamin A and carotene values of institutionalized mentally retarded subjects with and without Down's syndrome. *Journal of Mental Deficiency Research, 21*, 63.

Baselon, M., Paine, R.S., Cowie, V.A., Hunt, P., Houck, J.C., & Mahanand, D. (1976). Reversal of hypotonia in infants with Down's syndrome by administration of 5-hydroxytryptophan. *Lancet, 1*, 1130.

Beal, V.A. (1961). Dietary intake of individuals followed through infancy and childhood. *American Journal of Public Health, 51*, 1107.

Benda, C.E. (1969). *Down's syndrome: Mongolism and its management*. New York: Grune & Stratton.

Benda, C.E., & Mann, G.V. (1955). The serum cholesterol and lipoprotein levels in children. *Journal of Pediatrics, 46*, 49.

Bennett, F.C., McClelland, S., Kriesgsmann, E.A., Andrus, L.B., & Sells, C.J. (1983). Vitamin and mineral supplementation in Down's syndrome. *Pediatrics, 72* (5), 707–713.

Bjorksten, B., Back, O., Gustavson, K.H., Hallmans, B., HaggLof, B., & Tarnvik, A., (1980). Zinc and immune function in Down's syndrome. *Acta Paediatrics Scan, 69*, 183–187.

Bumbalo, T.S. (1964). Negative results: Treatment of Down syndrome with the "U" series. *Journal of the American Medical Association, 187*, 361.

Burgio, G.R., Ugazio, A., Nespoli, L., & Maccario, R. (1983). Down syndrome: A model of immunodeficiency. *Birth Defects* (original article Series), *19* (3), 325–327.

Calvert, S.D., Vivian, V.M., & Calvert, G.P. (1976). Dietary adequacy, feeding practices and eating behavior of children with Down's syndrome. *Journal of the American Diet Association, 69*, 152.

Chanowitz, J. et al. (1983). Thyroid and vitamin-mineral supplement fail to improve IQ of mentally retarded adults. *American Journal of Mental Deficiency, 90*, 217.

Chumlea, W.C., & Cronk, C.E. (1981). Overweight among children with Trisomy 21. *Journal of Mental Deficiency Research, 25*, 275–80.

Coleman, M. (Ed.). (1973). *Serotonin in Down's syndrome*. New York: Elsevier Publishers.

Costello, C., & Webber, A. (1976). White cell function in Down syndrome. *Clinical Genetics, 9*, 603–605.

Cronk, C.E. (1978). Growth of children with Down's syndrome: Birth to age three years. *Pediatrics, 61*, 564.

Cronk, C.E., & Chumlea, W.C. (1985). Is obesity a problem in Trisomy 21? *Trisomy 21* (1), 19–26.

Cronk, C.E., Crocker, A.C., Pueschel, S.M., Shea, A.M., Zackai, E., Pickens, G., & Reed, R.B. (1988). Growth charts for children with Down syndrome: 1 month to 18 years of age. *Pediatrics, 81*, 102.

Cronk, C.E., & Pueschel, S.M. (1984). Anthropometric studies. In S.M. Pueschel

(Ed.). *The young child with Down syndrome* (pp. 105–141). New York: Human Science Press.

Cullen, S.M., Cronk, C.E., Pueschel, S.M., Schnell, R.R., & Reed, R.B. (1981). Social development and feeding milestones of young Down syndrome children. *American Journal of Mental Deficiency, 85*, 410–415.

Culley, W.J., Goyal, K., Jolly, D.H., & Mertz, E.T. (1965). Caloric intake of children with Down's syndrome (Mongolism). *Journal of Pediatrics, 66*, 772–775.

Cutress, T.W., Mickelson, K.N.P., & Brown, R.H. (1976). Vitamin A absorption and periodontal disease in Trisomy G. *Journal of Mental Deficiency Research, 21*, 63.

Ellis, N.R., & Tomporowski, P.D. (1983). Vitamin-mineral supplements and intelligence of institutionalized mentally retarded adults. *American Journal of Mental Deficiency, 88*, 211–214.

Ellman, G., Schaefer, W.P., & Silverstein, L. (1984). Vitamin-mineral supplement fails to improve IQ of mentally retarded young adults. *American Journal of Mental Deficiency, 88*, Vol. 88, No. 6, 688–691.

Ershow, A.G. (1986). Growth in black and white children with Down syndrome. *American Journal of Mental Deficiency, 90*, 507–512.

Fomon, S. (1977). *Nutrition disorders of children—Prevention, screening, and follow-up*. DHEW (HSA), 77J–5104.

Frisancho, A.R. (1974). Triceps skinfold and upper arm assessment of nutritional status. *American Journal of Clinical Nutrition, 27*, 1077.

Frisancho, A.R. (1981). New norms of upper limb fat and muscle areas for assessment of nutrition status. *American Journal of Clinical Nutrition, 34*, 2540.

Geltz, R., & Geltz, E. (1984). *The food processor*. Salem, ESHA.

Gofman, J.W., DeLalla, O.F., Johnson, G., Kovich, E.L., Low, E., Piluso, D.L., Tandy, R.K.L., & Upham, R. (1962). Chemical elements of the blood of man. II: The levels of 66 chemical elements of Down's disease (Mongolism). *University of California Radiation Lab, 10211*, 69.

Giffith, A.W., & Behrman, J. (1965). Dark adaptation in Mongols. *Journal of Mental Deficiency Research, 9*, 164.

Harrell, R.F., Capp, R.H., Davis, D.K., Peerless, J., & Ravitz, L.R. (1981). Can nutritional supplements help mentally retarded children? An exploratory study. *Proceedings of the National Academy of Sciences, 78*, 574.

Hoshi, H., Ashizowa, K., & Ikeda, Y. (1979). Secular trend in growth in infants with Down's syndrome. *Human Biology, 51*, 289–297.

Jaswal, S., & Jaswal, I.J.S. (1981). An anthropometric study of body size in Down syndrome. *Indian Journal of Pediatrics, 48*, 81.

Jelliffe, D.B. (1966). *The assessment of the nutritional status of the community*. Geneva, Switzerland: World Health Organization (Monograph 53).

Johnson, C.L., Fulwood, R., Abraham, S., et al. (1981). Statistics Series II, No. 219.

Khan, A.J., Evans, H.E., Glass, L., Shin, Y.H., & Almonte, D. (1975). Defective neutrophil chemotaxis in patients with Down syndrome. *Journal of Pediatrics, 87*, 87–89.

Levin, S., Nir, E., & Mogilner, B.M. (1975). T-system immune deficiency in Down's syndrome. *Pediatrics, 56*, 123–126.

Matin, M.A., Sylvester, P.E., Edwards, D., & Dickerson, J.W.T. (1981). Vitamin zinc status in Down syndrome. *Journal of Mental Deficiency Research, 25*, 121–126.

Milunsky, A., Hackley, B.M., & Halsted, J.A. (1970). Plasma erythrocyte and leucocyte zinc levels in Down's syndrome. *Journal of Mental Deficiency Research, 14*, 99.

Nellhaus, G. (1968). Composite international and interracial graphs. *Pediatrics, 41*, 106.

Ogg, H.L. (1975). Oral pharyngeal development and evaluation. *Physical Therapy, 55*, 3.

Palmer, S. (1978a). Down's syndrome. In S. Palmer & S. Ekvall (Eds.), Pediatric nutrition in developmental disorders. Springfield, IL: Ches, C. Thomas.

Palmer, S. (1978b). Influence of vitamin A nutriture on the immune response: Findings in children with Down's syndrome. *International Journal of Vitamin Nutrition Research, 48*, 189.

Partington, M.W., MacDonald, M.R.A., & Tu, J.B. (1971). 5-hydroxytryptophan in Down's syndrome. *Dev Med Child Neurology, 13*, 362.

Pipes, P.L., & Holm, V.A. (1980). Feeding children with Down's syndrome. *Journal of American Dietetic Association, 77*, 277–281.

Pozsonyi, J., Gibson, D., & Zarfas, D.E. (1971). Growth deviations in handicapped children. *Clinical Pediatrics, 6*, 501.

Pozsonyi, J., & Lobb, H. (1967). Growth in mentally retarded children. *Journal of Pediatrics, 71*, 865.

Pueschel, S.M. (1984). The study population. In S.M. Pueschel (Ed.). *The young child with Down syndrome* (pp. 39–58). New York: Human Science Press.

Pueschel, S.M., & Pezzullo, J.C. (1985). Thyroid dysfunction in Down syndrome. *American Journal Diseases of Children, 139*, 636–639.

Pueschel, S.M., Reed, R.B., Cronk, C.E., & Goldstein, B.I. (1980). 5-hydroxy-tryptophan and pyridoxine: Their effect in young children with Down's syndrome. *American Journal of Diseases of Children, 134* (9), 838–844.

Rarick, G.L., & Seefeldt, V. (1974). Observations from longitudinal data on growth in stature and sitting height of children with Down's syndrome. *Journal of Mental Deficiency Research, 18*, 63.

Sharav, T., Collins, R.M., & Baab, P.J. (1988). Growth studies in infants and children with Down's Syndrome and elevated levels of thyrotropin. *American Journal of Diseases of Children, 142*, 1302.

Smith, C.F., Spiker, D., Peterson, C.P., Cicchetti, D., & Justine, P. (1984). Use of megadoses of vitamins with minerals in Down syndrome. *Journal of Pediatrics, 105* (2), 228–234.

Sobel, A.E., Strazzula, N., Sherman, B.S., Elkan, B., Morgenstern, S.W., Narius, N., & Kerisel, A. (1958). Vitamin A absorption and other blood composition studies in mongolism. *American Journal of Mental Deficiency, 62*, 324.

Stedman, D.J., & Eichorn, D.H. (1964). Comparison of the growth and development of institutionalized and home-reared mongoloids during infancy and early child-hood. *American Journal of Mental Deficiency, 69*, 391.

Tu, J.B., & Zellweger, H. (1965). Blood serotonin deficiency in Down's syndrome. *Lancet, 2* (415), 715–716.

Turkel, H. (1975). Medical amelioration of Down syndrome incorporating the orthomolecular approach. *Journal of Orthomolecul Psych, 4*, 102.

Walker, G.M. (1955). Nutrition in mentally deficient children. *Journal of American Dietetic Association, 31*, 495.

Weathers, C. (1983). Effects of nutritional supplementation on IQ and certain other variables associated with Down syndrome. *American Journal of Mental Deficiency, 88*, 214–217.

Weise, P., Koch, R., Shaw, K.N.F., & Rosenfeld, M.J. (1974). The use of 5-HTP in the treatment of Down's syndrome. *Pediatrics, 54*, 165.

White, D., & Kaplitz, S.E. (1964). Treatment of Down syndrome with a vitamin-mineral hormonal preparation. *International Copenhagen Congress: Scientific study of mental retardation, 1*, 224.

10
Developmental Assessment

MARTY NOVAK HOFFMAN AND RUTH ZEMKE

Introduction

There are several well standardized tools to measure children's development including Gesell Developmental Schedules and the Bayley Scales of Infant Development (BSID) (Eiper & Azen, 1978). However, only a small body of information on the scores of children with Down syndrome exists that can be used as a basis for comparison with other children. The literature has shown that there is a wide range of abilities in children with Down syndrome and, therefore a wide range of performance ratings on developmental instruments (LaVeck & Brehm, 1978).

In studies reviewed, 88 children made up the largest sample, 22 the smallest. Furthermore, studies yield contradicting results. For example, Zausmer and Shea (1984) conclude that motor development in Down syndrome follows a normal progression, while other studies conclude it does not (Carr, 1975; Morss, 1983; Schnell, 1984; Silverstein, Legutki et al., 1982).

Studies have also been completed on the performance on the BSID of children with Down syndrome (Carr, 1970; Schnell, 1984). However, even with these specific data, conflicting information continues to be gathered regarding developmental expectations for these children. Further examination of development in children with Down syndrome, of evaluation tools, and of treatment programs is needed.

Current developmental assessment tools have usually been standardized on children without disabilities, even though many of these tools are also used to assess children who have disabilities. Because of this, certain potential biases exist in testing, especially when the tests are used in an attempt to compare children with handicaps to normative data on children without handicaps. According to LaGrow and Prochnow-LaGrow (1985), biases exist in assessments when groups or populations of children score consistently lower than predicted from the norms of the test. This invariably happens when testing children with Down syndrome; in fact, a consistent lower score is frequently expected, reflecting the expectation of lower mental and physical functions associated with the diagnosis of Down syndrome. Legal requirements for nondiscriminatory testing, however, include the use of tools that accurately reflect children's skills and aptitudes, rather than measure the level of the disability (LaGrow & Prochnow-LaGrow, 1985).

Using appropriate normative data is not the only important issue in testing children with Down syndrome. The type of score used is also important. Comparisons are usually made of a child's score to the tool's standard score. This generally identifies how that child is performing relative to a sample of children intended to reflect the general population of that age group.

Standard scores are frequently converted to intelligence quotients and age equivalent scores to give further meaning to the score. This is especially true with exceptional children who frequently score so low that meaning in the standard score is lost. Bayley (1969) advocates the use of age equivalents rather than the computation of an intelligence quotient. Intelligence quotients are computed by dividing the mental age score by the child's chronological age. Bayley (1969) states that computation of intelligence quotients should not be done as "there is no evidence to support interpretation of a figure of this kind from the BSID."

Age equivalents, although useful, also have limitations. Disadvantages are identified by Angoff (1984), who concludes that there is a certain amount of ambiguity in age equivalents. Angoff explains that two comparison regression lines exist in a correlation less than equal. In correlating age with test performance, the two regression lines identified were regression of age on test performance and regression of test performance for age. The translation of the test score into age equivalents could be based on either one of these lines, so that for the same test score two different ages could be given. The lower the correlation between the age and test performance, the greater the discrepancy between the two will be.

Lastly, in indentifying a specific "age" at which a child is said to be functioning, based on test performance, one cannot say the child is acting typically for the age. Many skills are present at a given age, and a test can measure only a sample of them. Thus, an age equivalent cannot mean that all aspects of a child's behavior are truly and totally age appropriate (Angoff, 1984). However, although age equivalents have limitations, they also provide concrete feedback about a child's performance. If age equivalents are used with a cautionary explanation of their limitations, they are beneficial to understanding the overall development of the child.

The BSID was designed to provide a tool for measurement of the development of infants from the age of 2 to 30 months, for both clinical and research purposes. There are three sections to the BSID: the mental scale, the psychomotor scale, and the infant behavior record.

Scoring of the BSID is initially recorded as either success or failure on each item of the mental and psychomotor scale. The infant behavior record is intended for subjective, qualitative observations while testing. Basal and ceiling levels can then be established. The basal level is the item preceding the first failure. The ceiling level is the item representing the last success. A raw score for each scale is computed by adding the total number of items passed, including all items below the basal level. The use of the tables in the testing manual allows conversion of a raw score into an age equivalent or developmental age, a mental developmental index score, and a psychomotor developmental index score. Both of these index scores are normalized standard scores, which Bayley states have "the same numerical characteristics" as intelligent quotients (Bayley, 1969).

The BSID has been used in many of the research projects in child development (Carr, 1975; Harris, 1981; LaVeck & LaVeck, 1977; Schnell, 1984). It has further been recommended as the tool of choice for developmental evaluations by Eiper and Azen (1978). This, in addition to its base in developmental theory, makes the BSID ideal for this study and for the purposes of the program under study. With strong reliability and standardization information with normal children, the BSID lends itself to development for other populations, namely, children with Down syndrome for identification and comparison. In addition, the BSID is commonly used with children who have Down syndrome as the instrument of choice for research purposes because the Gesell developmental schedule may overestimate the developmental level in children with developmental delay because it relies on report more than observation (Eiper & Azen, 1978).

Schnell (1984) used the Pearson product-moment correlation for a comparison of each scale of the BSID with itself across time, and repeated measures for comparison between the two scales. All correlation coefficients were significant at the 0.01 level. A correlation between the immediate past score and the present score on the BSID mental scales became progressively larger, reaching a peak at 18 months and not changing significantly thereafter. Approximately 70% of the variance was common between the mental scores. On the BSID psychomotor scales, the correlation between the immediate past score and the present score reached its height at 24 months, accounting for 69% of the variance. Correlations between the mental and psychomotor scales increased until 18 months, which accounted for approximately 46% of the variance and slightly decreased to 36 months.

Schnell (1984) further reported that the correlations of the mental and psychomotor scales for normal children held a lesser relationship than those for children with Down syndrome. For children with Down syndrome the psychomotor scale's predictability of the mental scale at 36 months progressively increased from 6 to 36 months, accounting for 35% of the variance. the mental scale's predictability of the psychomotor scale performance at 36 months accounted for 42% of the variance at 18 to 24 months, then decreased 35% at 36 months.

Past Studies of Down Syndrome

BSID scores of children with Down syndrome who had mild congenital heart disease, were compared by Schnell with those who had moderate to severe cardiac problems. The differences between the two groups were significant at the 0.05 level by a t-test at the 12-, 18-, 24-, and 36-month levels in motor formance, but only at the 12-month level in mental performance. Differences between the children with mild conditions and children with moderate and severe cardiac conditions were thought to be caused by the requirement of walking in the motor scale. The Down syndrome children with moderate to severe cardiac problems probably were walking much later than those without cardiac problems, as children with severe cardiac problems have poor circulation and are generally more lethargic (Cunningham, 1982; Schnell, 1984).

Independent of the BSID, children with Down syndrome were also grouped by ratings of muscle tone. They were divided into two groups, those with poor muscle tone and those with good muscle tone. For this analysis, the children with moderate and severe cardiac deficiencies were excluded. Differences between means on the psychomotor scale with a one-way analysis of variance were significant at the 0.05 level or less, beginning with the 12-month age group. On the mental scale, a 0.3-month difference between groups was noted at the 6-month level, increasing to a 3.7-month difference at the 36-month level. On the psychomotor scale, the 6-month level was a 0.9-month difference increasing to a 4.2-month difference at the 36-month level (Schnell, 1984).

Schnell (1984) concluded that the data obtained indicate children with Down syndrome display a linear development as reflected by scores on the mental scale (see Appendix 6). Linear development means that with a regular increase in chronological age there will be a regular increase in developmental age. On the psychomotor scale, however, deceleration with age was noted in the developmental quotients with age. Correlations between the mental and psychomotor scales indicate a stronger relationship between the two scales for children with Down syndrome than for other children. He also concludes that the BSID becomes increasingly better at predicting future scores of children with Down syndrome on that scale. The problems secondary to Down syndrome, such as cardiac conditions and muscle tone, were shown to affect development. The effect was especially apparent in performance on the psychomotor scale.

Carr (1970) completed a longitudinal study of 54 children with Down syndrome between the ages of 6 weeks and 2 years. Each child was tested at 6 weeks, 6 months, 10 months, 15 months, and 2 years. Carr (1970) noted a general decline in developmental quotients on both the mental and motor scales of the BSID from birth until 10 months. The decline in both developmental quotients became more gradual to 24 months, indicating lags in development, which decelerated with age. These findings concur with those previously cited by Schnell (1984), in that both studies note a decrease in scores with age. The studies differ, however, for Schnell notes an almost linear relationship with the decrease in performance and age. Carr's study indicates that there was not a linear relationship for that sample, but rather the decrease became less with increasing age.

Comparisons were made by Schneider and Brannen (1984) between the BSID and the revised Gesell developmental schedules in a cross-sectional study of 20 children with Down syndrome between the ages of 6 and 36 months. Results indicated that the mean motor deficit was significantly greater than the mean mental deficit in both instruments. This supports the findings of earlier studies (LaVeck & LaVeck, 1977). The mental and motor discrepancy also corresponded positively with chronological age in both scales, with motor deficits increasing at a faster rate. There were no differences between scores of males and females.

According to Carr (1970), children with Down syndrome showed more fluctuations on repeated measures in scores on the BSID than a control group. Carr found 62% of the scores fluctuated between test and retest in the children with Down syndrome compared to 40% in the control group. Eighty-three percent of the score fluctuations in the control group were less than 30 points with none being over 40. Fifty-one percent of the score fluctuations in the Down syndrome group were below 30 points; however, 27% of the Down syndrome group scores were over 40 points (Carr, 1970). With increased fluctuations on test-retest, there is a possibility that children with Down syndrome would score differently on retesting. However, Schnell (1984) concludes that the BSID has increasingly better predictability of future scores on the scale with increasing age. This is in opposition to Carr's conclusions, discussed earlier.

In summary, researchers have used the BSID with children with Down syndrome to measure development. Data show that there is a steady, marked decline in the scores to a certain age, and then the decline becomes more gradual. Further conclusions indicate higher correlations between the mental and psychomotor scales for children with Down syndrome than for normal children, and that sex differences are not significant. Cardiac problems are significant in the performance of several groups on the psychomotor scale, but in only one age group on the mental scale. Lastly, motor deficiencies are noted to be greater than mental deficiencies with increasing age.

Methods

For approximately 18 months, between 1984 and 1986, the City of Hope National Medical Centre in Duarte, California, conducted a comprehensive evaluation program for children of all ages with diagnosis of Down syndrome. Parents were referred to the program by physicians, regional centers, and other parents of children with Down syndrome. The only criterion for admission was the diagnosis of Down syndrome.

Subjects included in the study reported in this chapter were children with Down syndrome between the ages of 2 and 30 months. Other children older than 30 months were evaluated with the BSID in this program but are not included in this discussion. These children ($n = 66$ for the psychomotor scale,

$n = 76$ for the mental scale) were seen at the City of Hope for evaluation by staff, including occupational therapists and a psychologist, using the BSID.

The main goal was to provide mean developmental ages for children with Down syndrome between the ages of 2 months and 30 months. By having this information, professionals working on this population could refer to these local norms to compare their patients developmental age on the Bayley Scales of Infant Development. This comparison would show whether the tested child with Down syndrome is scoring above or below the mean developmental age for that child's chronological age group of children with Down syndrome. The raw scores necessary to derive these developmental ages were also included, as the raw scores, not the developmental ages, are actually the local norms.

Data Collection and Analysis

All of the children with Down syndrome referred to the program were seen by psychologists and occupational therapists.

When children were seen for evaluation, team conferences were held so that results from all disciplines could be reported. Information on each child, inclusive of the parental report of demographics and testing results, were entered into a computer (IBM PC/XT). Thus, the data for this study were collected by obtaining demographic information, raw scores, and developmental ages on the mental and psychomotor scales of the BSID for each of the children with DS from the existing computer data base (mental index scores and psychomotor index scores were calculated from the raw score).

The sample was categorized by the chronological age groups generally following the same division that was used for the normative sample of the Bayley Scales of Infant Development.

That is, for infants between the ages of 2 months and 6 months, one month intervals were used (forming 5 age groups, 2, 3, 4, 5 and 6 months). For infants between the ages of 7 months and 12 months, 2 month intervals were used (3 age groups of 7–8, 9–10, and 11–12 months). Three month intervals for children between the ages of 12 months and 30 months were used (forming 6 age groups consisting of 13–15, 16–18, 19–21, 22–24, 25–27, and 28–30 months). Age was calculated by breaking 15 days beyond each month such that if children were 3 months and 15 days, they were placed in the 3 month age group; on the other hand, if they were 3 months and 16 days, they were placed in the 4 month age group.

Results

A total of 78 children with Down syndrome were tested on the BSID (see Appendix 7). Of the 78 children, 64 were tested with both the mental and the psychomotor scales. A total of 76 children were tested on the mental scale, with 12 tested on the mental scale exclusively (Appendix 7). A total of 66 children were tested on the psychomotor scale, with two of those children tested by the psychomotor scale exclusively.

The ratio of males to females in the sample was slightly less than one to one; of 78 children, 41 were female and 37 were male. The ratio of children tested for each scale did not appear different from that of the total sample. The ages of the children in the total sample ranged from 2 to 30 months, with a mean of 13.5 and a standard deviation of 8.3.

There was essentially the same distribution of type of Down syndrome when comparing the total sample to those children tested on the psychomotor scale and the mental scale. Of the children tested, all were diagnosed as having trisomy 21, 4 children had translocation, and 2 children were mosaic. The data from this study follows a fairly normal distribution for type of Down syndrome. That is, the majority of children with Down syndrome will have Trisomy 21, while approximately 2 to 5% of children will have Down syndrome due to mosaic or a translocation.

All other demographic information for the sample whose Bayley scores are reported in this chapter did not differ significantly from the entire population described in Appendix I.

The results for each subject are listed in Appendix 5, which includes the raw scores, developmental ages, and index score for each of the scales. The index score (a standard score) was calculated, except for those children who scored lower than three standard deviations below the mean. In those cases, the index score was identified as > -3 SD. Appendices 8 and 9 describe the categorization of the chronological age groups for each scale. Means and standard deviations were included for the raw scores and developmental ages for each of the age groups.

The mean raw score increases in each chronolgical age group with few exceptions. At the 4 month age group in both the mental and the psychomotor scores there is a decrease in the mean raw score and mean developmental age. As there were only two children tested for the psychomotor scale and three for the mental scale these means most likely reflect the low score for one individual, subject 10 (see Appendices 8 and 9). Another exception is at 25–27 months where only one subject was tested. This child scored low on the psychomotor scale but relatively as expected on the mental scale (subject 68 in Appendices 8 and 9). At 28–30 months there is a decrease in the mental raw scores and developmental ages. This is probably due to the very low scores of subjects 76 and 77 (Appendices 8 and 9). These two subjects also scored very low on the psychomotor scale, however the effect did not seem as dramatic as in the mental scale at this age group due to the already low performance at the 25–27 months age group.

The mean raw scores and developmental ages for the children tested with Down syndrome essentially follow a normal developmental pattern showing increases in mean scores with increasing chronological ages. There were some exceptions, as in certain cases there were either few subjects or one very low score which affected the means for an age group.

A Spearman rank-order correlation coefficient (rho) was calculated and yielded a high correlation between the two scales, even when adjusted for age (rho = .9124). A high correlation is also found in the literature between the two scales for children with Down syndrome. These correlations, both from the literature and this study, are higher than that established in the normative data for the BSID.

Results indicate that psychomotor development is consistently slower than mental development. Results also supported previous studies identified in the literature review that show a deceleration with age in both areas of development.

Regression lines were calculated for both scales to identify a change in the rate of development with increasing chronological age. For each scale a regression line was formed for those children in the < 10–12-month age group, and for those children > 12 months. There was a significant change in the rate of development between the children up to one year and those older than one year, in both the mental and psychomotor scales ($p < 0.05$) with mental performance being consistently better than psychomotor performance throughout all ages.

Discussion

Children with Down syndrome are frequently seen in child developmental clinics by medical and educational professions. These children may have varying types and degrees of disabilities, including some form of mental and developmental retardation, muscular hypotonia, and the strong possibility of congenital heart disease of varying severity (Buckley, 1984; Cunningham, 1982; Menkes, 1980).

The development of children with Down syndrome is known to occur with greater variability and at a much slower rate than that of other children. In addition, it has been suggested that developmental patterns in children with Down syndrome might also be different from those of children with other disabilities, although current literature offers conflicting views (Cunningham, 1982, Morss, 1983). Whether slow or different, studies indicate that mental skills are generally better than motor skills, and that there is a deceleration in development with increasing chronological age (Carr, 1975; Schnell, 1982). However, results of studies differ as the the rate of this change. Schnell (1984) noted a sharp deceleration in motor development in children with Down syndrome. As tested on the BSID, the children in Schnell's study were performing at 67% of normal levels at 6 months, and at 53% at 36 months. In contrast, testing with the BSID, Carr (1970) noted a general decline from normal performance in birth to 10 months, with the decline continuing at a lesser rate to 24 months. These authors demonstrated further conflicting results. Schnell (1984) demonstrated that children with Down syndrome display a linear development (with regular increases in chronological age there were regular increases in developmental age). Carr (1970) did not find the same linear relationship, but rather found a decrease in development, the rate of which became less with increasing chronological age. Thus, current research offers conflicting information about the development of children with Down syndrome.

One conclusion based on the results of our study and a review of the literature was that, in general, the development of children with Down syndrome is linear. That is, their development progresses with increasing chronological age. However, an exact description of this linear relationship varies, both in this study and studies reported in the literature. Schnell (1984) notes a deceleration of development with age in performance on the psychomotor scale, but not on the mental scale; that is, the linear relationship differs between the two scales. Schnell (1984) did not find deceleration in the mental scale scores with increasing age. Carr (1970) found that scores of both the mental and psychomotor scales reflect a deceleration in development, with the decrease becoming less with increasing age. That is, the linear relationship was the same between the two scales, but changed with the increasing chronological age.

In this study there was a general deceleration of development performance on the mental and psychomotor scales. Also, the rate of the deceleration differs with age. Carr (1970) noted a general decline from birth to 10 months; from 10 to 24 months the decline became more gradual. Our study demonstrated that the decline became greater for those children in the sample older than 12 months. The children with Down syndrome in this sample were demonstrating poorer performance (relative to the norms) with increasing age. Schnell (1984) noted decreasing results with increasing chronolgical age, but only in the psychomotor scale.

From the results of the regression lines calculated it was supported that the rate of development changed in the performance on both the mental and psychomotor scales with increasing chronological age. On the mental scale the children < 10–12 months performed at 79% of the level of children without disabilities, and the children > 12 months performed at 55%. This differs with Schnell's (1984) finding that on the mental scale children with Down syndrome between 6 to 36 months chronologically performed between 55–58%, just slightly lower than the results from this study. Schnell (1984) further documented that children at 36 months chronologically performed at 53% which is just slightly lower than the results from this study for children up to 30 months of age.

Results of our study indicate that there is a high correlation between the mental and psychomotor scales for the sample of children with Down syndrome. It is not so high that one would interpret this correlation as due to any overriding factor measured by both scales to the detriment of each scale's uniqueness. However, the standardization sample did not account for the performance of children with Down syndrome. The correlation established in this study of children with Down syndrome was higher than for the standardization sample. Schnell (1984) also found a higher correlation between

A Spearman rank-order correlation coefficient (rho) was calculated and yielded a high correlation between the two scales, even when adjusted for age (rho = .9124). A high correlation is also found in the literature between the two scales for children with Down syndrome. These correlations, both from the literature and this study, are higher than that established in the normative data for the BSID.

Results indicate that psychomotor development is consistently slower than mental development. Results also supported previous studies identified in the literature review that show a deceleration with age in both areas of development.

Regression lines were calculated for both scales to identify a change in the rate of development with increasing chronological age. For each scale a regression line was formed for those children in the < 10–12-month age group, and for those children > 12 months. There was a significant change in the rate of development between the children up to one year and those older than one year, in both the mental and psychomotor scales ($p < 0.05$) with mental performance being consistently better than psychomotor performance throughout all ages.

Discussion

Children with Down syndrome are frequently seen in child developmental clinics by medical and educational professions. These children may have varying types and degrees of disabilities, including some form of mental and developmental retardation, muscular hypotonia, and the strong possibility of congenital heart disease of varying severity (Buckley, 1984; Cunningham, 1982; Menkes, 1980).

The development of children with Down syndrome is known to occur with greater variability and at a much slower rate than that of other children. In addition, it has been suggested that developmental patterns in children with Down syndrome might also be different from those of children with other disabilities, although current literature offers conflicting views (Cunningham, 1982, Morss, 1983). Whether slow or different, studies indicate that mental skills are generally better than motor skills, and that there is a deceleration in development with increasing chronological age (Carr, 1975; Schnell, 1982). However, results of studies differ as the the rate of this change. Schnell (1984) noted a sharp deceleration in motor development in children with Down syndrome. As tested on the BSID, the children in Schnell's study were performing at 67% of normal levels at 6 months, and at 53% at 36 months. In contrast, testing with the BSID, Carr (1970) noted a general decline from normal performance in birth to 10 months, with the decline continuing at a lesser rate to 24 months. These authors demonstrated further conflicting results. Schnell (1984) demonstrated that children with Down syndrome display a linear development (with regular increases in chronological age there were regular increases in developmental age). Carr (1970) did not find the results of this design included all ages but grouped in small clusters. The discrepancy between Schnell's (1984) results and the results of our study could be due to the lower ages included in a specific age group. For example, Schnell tested all children at exactly 30 months. This study included children between the ages of 28 and 30 months. Although there are some differences at the three age groups, the findings from this cross-sectional design are fairly consistent with those of Schnell, who used a longitudinal design. Thus, a cross-sectional design for describing longitudinal patterns in performance can be considered adequate, although not optimal.

From the results of our study and Schnell's (1984) work, one can conclude that the expected performance on the psychomotor scale of children with Down syndrome when compared to non–Down syndrome children decreases with increasing chronological age. One would expect that motor development in a child with Down syndrome would be a progression in motor skills with increasing chronological age but that this progression would slow as the child became older.

Looking only at the results of this study, the performance on the mental scale of children with Down syndrome, when compared to children without Down syndrome, also decreases with increasing chronological age. This suggests expectations for mental development in a child with Down syndrome would be for a progression of cognitive skills with increasing chronological age, but that this progression would slow as the child became older, as would motor development, but to a lesser degree. As stated previously, mental skills are generally better than motor skills. This conclusion is in contrast to Schnell's (1984) statement that mental performance stays constant with increasing chronological age and Carr's (1970) statement of less decrease with increasing chronolgical age.

Our results also were very similar to Schnell's results when comparing mean developmental age scores, even though this study was completed cross sectionally and Schnell's study was completed longitudinally. The similarities between the two studies are extremely important as the likenesses give support for the results even when considering potential errors in design. These similarities also indicate that the samples of children with Down syndrome were probably very similar for both studies. A small sample size for each age group is a definite limitation to our study, but with the similarities of the mean scores to Schnell's results, the severity of this limitation is lessened, possibly even to the point of being negligible. Unfortunately, Schnell did not complete mean developmental ages for as many age groups as this study so that comparison can only be made to a few age groups. Nevertheless, the age groups that can be compared are similar.

Summary

As measured on the BSID, the developmental profile of children with Down syndrome is of greater variability and slower rate than that of non-Down syndrome children. Mental skills in children with this syndrome are generally better than motor skills with a deceleration in both areas of development with increasing chronological age. In general, the development of children with Down syndrome is linear with developmental progress occurring with increasing chronological age. The exact description of this linear relationship varies from study to study.

In general, deceleration of developmental performance in Down syndrome children occurs in both the mental and psychomotor areas. This study demonstrates that the decline is greatest for those children older than 12 months of age. On the mental scale Down syndrome children less than 10 to 12 months performed at 79% of the level of children without Down syndrome, and children greater than 12 months of age, 55%. These children performed consistently higher on the mental scale of the BSID in comparison to the psychomotor scale, with a high correlation between the mental and psychomotor scales. Cardiac problems did not significantly affect performance on either the mental or psychomotor scales.

This study was completed to provide professionals with specific age group data for children with Down Syndrome (see also Appendixes 8 and 9). By providing the mean raw scores and mean developmental ages, professionals using the Bayley Scales of Infant Development can refer to these in their evaluation process. Some age groups have limited use due to their very small size but overall it is hoped that these groups will be a useful reference tool.

References

Angoff, W. (1984). *Scales, norms, and equivalent scores.* Princeton, NJ: Educational Testing Service.

Bayley, N. (1969). *Bayley scales of infant development.* New York: The Psychological Corp.

Buckley, L. (1984). Cardiac assessments. In S. Pueschel (Ed.), *The young child with Down syndrome* (pp. 351–664). New York: Human Sciences Press.

Carr, J. (1970). Mental and motor development in young Mongol children. *Journal of Mental Deficiency Research, 14* (31), 205–220.

Carr, J. (1975). *Young children with Down's syndrome.* London: Butterworths.

Cunningham, C. (1982). *Down's syndrome: An introduction for parents.* London: Souvenir Press.

Eiper, D.S., & Azen, S.P. (1978). A comparison of two developmental instruments in evaluating children with Down's syndrome. *Physical Therapy, 58* (9), 1066–1069.

Harris, S. (1981). Relationship of mental and motor development of Down's syndrome infants. *Phys Occup Ther in Pediatr, 1*, 13–18.

LaGrow, S., & Prochnow-LaGrow, J. (1985). Consideration of bias in the assessment and placement process of exceptional children. In A. Rotatori & R. Fox (Eds.), *Assessment for regular and special education teachers.* Austin, TX: Pro-Ed, Inc.

LaVeck, B., & Brehm, S.S. (1978). Individual variability among children with Down's syndrome. *Mental Retardation, 16* (2), 135–137.

LaVeck, B., & LaVeck, G.D. (1977). Sex differences in development among young children with Down's syndrome. *Journal of Pediatrics, 91* (5), 767–769.

Menkes, J. (1980). *Child neurology*, (2d ed.). Philadelphia: Lea & Febiger.

Morss, R.J. (1983). Cognitive development in the Down's syndrome infant: Slow or different? *Brit Jour of Educ Psych, 53* (1), 40–47.

Schneider, J., & Brannen, E. (1984). A comparison of two developmental evaluation tools used to assess children with Down's syndrome. *Phys and Occup Ther in Pediatr, 4*, 19–29.

Schnell, R. (1984). Psychomotor development. In S. Pueschel (Ed.), *The young child with Down syndrome*. New York: Human Sciences Press.

Silverstein, A.B., Legutki, G., Friedman, S.L., & Takayama, D.L. (1982). Performance of Down syndrome individuals on the Stanford-Binet intelligence scale. *American Journal of Mental Deficiency, 86* (5), 548–551.

Zausmer, E., & Shea, A. (1984). Motor development. In S. Pueschel (Ed.), *The young child with Down syndrome* (p. 143). New York: Human Sciences Press.

11
P300 Latency and Cognitive Ability

Stacy L. Schantz and Warren S. Brown

Introduction

From infancy, cognitive deficiencies are apparent in all individuals with Down syndrome (Morss, 1983). The mean IQ for children with this syndrome is approximately 40–50, but varies widely from severely retarded (IQ around 10) to low-normal (IQ around 90) intelligence (Connolly, 1978). Along with the wide range of abilities found in Down Syndrome, instability of the measures of cognitive performance is characteristic (Morss, 1983). Current tests of cognitive functioning do not provide for good generalizability across levels of development in children with Down syndrome (Hartley, 1986). The difficulty in finding tests of mental ability appropriate for the individual with this syndrome is perhaps the source of conflicting reports about the abilities of Down syndrome populations. Therefore, developmental norms on tests of general mental ability are needed, norms that are applicable to individuals with a wide range of cognitive abilities and that are not greatly affected by a lack of cooperation.

The cause of lowered cognitive abilities in Down syndrome is unknown but may be related to anatomical differences in the brains of these individuals, including smaller brainstem and cerebellar structures than in the normal population, generalized cellular agenesis, fibrillary gliosis of cortical neurons, incomplete myelination, impaired development of cortical U-fibers, and a smaller and maldeveloped hippocampus (Sylvester, 1983). The average brain weight in children with Down syndrome is less than that of other children (Crome & Stern, 1972).

Event-Related Potentials and Cognitive Ability in Down Syndrome

One approach to a better understanding of information processing in Down syndrome is the use of event-related EEG potentials (ERPs) (Callner et al., 1978; Gliddon et al., 1975; Lincoln et al., 1985; Squires et al., 1979). Of particular interest in recent studies has been the latency of ERP components, particularly the P300 (Lincoln et al., 1985; Squires et al., 1979). The P300 is a long-latency, "endogenous" component of the ERP that reflects neural responses associated with the higher mental processes of stimulus recognition, evaluation and categorization (Pritchard, 1981). The latency of the P300 is a measure of the time taken by the brain to sufficiently categorize a stimulus to a relevant task, independent of any motor or verbal responses that may also be required (Duncan-Johnson, 1981; Kutas, McCarthy, & Donchin, 1977; McCarthy & Donchin, 1981).

P300 latency changes in a systematic way with the aging process in normal individuals. Longer latency values are recorded for younger children (6–14 years), with the P300 decreasing progressively during development and stabilizing at approximately 300 msec at about 15 years of age (Courchesne, 1977, 1978). A slower age-related increase in latency (about 1 msec per yr) occurs throughout adulthood (Brown et al., 1983; Goodin et al., 1978).

P300 latency has also been found useful as a means of evaluating cognitive functioning for patients with dementing brain disease, or for revealing subtle changes in cognitive function due to other medical disorders and/or treatments (Brown et al., 1982; Marsh et al., 1986; Squires et al., 1980). Squires et al. (1980) found, for example, that P300 latency correlated with mental status in patients with disorders affecting the nervous system. They suggest P300 latency may be a sensitive means for evaluating changes in cognitive functioning resulting from neurological dysfunction. Marsh et al. (manuscript in preparation) have recently shown that: (1) even in the very early stages of Alzheimer's dementia, normal and demented individuals can be discriminated using P300 latency; and (2) there is a strong correlation between P300 latency prolongation and decrease in the metabolic activity of the parietal cortex as revealed by PET scan.

P300 latency has also proven valuable in discriminating children with different cognitive abilities (Heukrodt et al., 1988; Rothenberger & Baschek, 1982). Heukrodt et al. (1988) found significant differences in P300 between children who had recovered from acute lymphoblastic leukemia and normal children. P300 latency correlated significantly with children's intelligence scores on the Weschler Intelligence Scales for Children ($r = -0.52$ to -0.72), and with the Wide Range Achievement Scales ($r = -0.44$ to -0.49). Thus, the current literature on the P300 strongly supports its utility as an objective, noninvasive means of evaluating cognitive functioning for a variety of subject populations.

Down syndrome children have been shown to have abnormal ERPS. Components earlier than the P300 are generally less variable, larger in amplitude, and somewhat longer in latency (Callner & Dustman, 1975; Callner et al., 1978; also see Straumanis et al., 1973; Yellin et al. 1980, regarding latency). Callner et al. (1978) and others have speculated that the differences in the early ERP components are due to deficits in central inhibition or abnormalities in neuronal excitability in Down syndrome individuals.

A few investigators have examined later ERP wave components such as the P300 in persons with Down syndrome (Galbraith et al., 1979; Squires et al., 1979 and Lincoln et al., 1985). Squires et al. (1979) found that Down syndrome children had smaller amplitude and longer latency P300s than normal subjects. Similarly, Lincoln et al. (1985) found P300 latency was longer by approximately 50 msec in the Down syndrome population when they were compared to chronological-age-matched normal controls. When they were compared to mental age matched controls, the Down syndrome subjects had shorter P300 latencies. Lincoln et al. (1985) see the Down syndrome population as not merely slower but different from other children in their brain responses and organization. Given the similarities recently demonstrated between Alzheimer disease and Down syndrome (Kolata, 1985; Wisniewski, Howe, Williams, & Wisniewski, 1978), it is not surprising that Down syndrome patients, like those with Alzheimer disease, have prolonged P300 latencies.

In summary, as with other patients with lowered mental status, Down syndrome subjects have longer latency P300 components. Given the high correlation found in previous studies between P300 latency and measures of mental status in neurologically impaired adults (Squires et al., 1980), and between P300 latency and the intellectual abilities of learning disordered children (Heukrodt et al., 1988), it is conceivable that P300 latency may be useful as a tool in the assessment of the cognitive abilities of individual children with Down syndrome. P300 latency may index the integrity of neural systems critical to cognitive, linguistic, and social functioning of individuals with this syndrome.

Thus, studies designed to assess the latency of the P300 component of the auditory ERP as an index of cognitive ability in children with Down syndrome and age-matched normals controls may show P300 to be a useful assessment tool. P300 latency may not only account for a large percentage of the difference in cognitive ability between subjects with and without Down syndrome, but also a large percentage of the variance in cognitive ability within the Down syndrome group.

A Study of P300 Latency and Cognitive Ability in Down Syndrome

Fifteen subjects with Down syndrome and 16 non-Down syndrome children between 5 and 19 years of age were evaluated to determine their P300 latencies in response to an auditory "odd-ball" tones detection task. Subjects were asked merely to raise a finger every time they recognized the rare tone. ERPs were recorded and averaged in response to the 32 rare tones and the 32 frequents (of a total of 128 frequent tones) that preceded the rares. Down syndrome subjects were also administered the following tests of intellectual ability and social competency: the McCarthy Scales for Children's Abilities, the Vineland Adaptive Behavior Scale, the Peabody Picture Vocabulary Test,

TABLE 11.1. Subject characteristics.

	Down syndrome		Non-Down syndrome	
	X	Range	X	Range
Sex (males/females)	7/8		7/9	
Age (months)	126	62–229	121	80–228
VMA (months)	57	15–96	146	79–396
PMA (months)	54	15–70	139	87–174
P300 latency	470	360–650	387	260–656

TABLE 11.2. Regression of P300 latency and mental ability.

Combined	
VMA	$r=-0.46$, $p<0.01$
PMA	$r=-0.52$, $p<0.01$
Non-Down syndrome	
VMA	$r=-0.39$, $p=0.12$
PMA	$r=-0.43$, $p=0.07$
Down syndrome	
VMA	$r=0.22$, $p=0.45$
PMA	$r=0.07$, $p=0.81$

and the Developmental Test of Visual Motor Integration (Beery). Non-Down syndrome children were administered the Developmental Test of Visual Motor Integration (Beery), and the Peabody Picture Vocabulary Test.

Results

As with previous studies of P300 latencies in subjects with Down syndrome, a significant latency difference was found between Down syndrome and non-Down syndrome children. The mean latency for the Down syndrome group was 83 msec longer than that of the non-Down syndrome children ($p<0.01$).

Regression analysis was performed to determine the correlation between P300 latency and verbal and performance mental ages in both groups individually as well as together. When the data from the Down syndrome and non-Down syndrome groups were combined, significant correlations were found for both performance mental age (PMA) and verbal mental age (VMA: see Table 11.2). However, with the Down syndrome group there was no significant association between the latency of the P300 component and verbal or performance ability as measured by the Peabody, Beery, or McCarthy tests. P300 latency also was not found to correlate significantly with either the McCarthy subtests of memory or general cognitive index or with the Vineland tests of communication, socialization, or absolute behavior composite.

Although the Down syndrome group had a larger mean P300 amplitude than the non-Down syndrome children, these differences were not significant. The Down syndrome group had particularly large P300 amplitude over frontal scalp areas, but differences in P300 amplitude scalp distribution were not significant, nor was scalp distribution correlated with cognitive ability.

Discussion and Conclusions: P300 as an Assessment Tool in Down Syndrome

P300 latency was again shown to be longer for children with Down syndrome. When the children and the control subjects were considered together, P300 latency correlated significantly with measures of PIQ and VIQ. That these correlations with cognitive ability were primarily reflective of the P300 latency and IQ differences between the Down syndrome and non-Down syndrome control groups is suggested by the lack of significant correlation within groups between the P300 measures and mental and social ability. Although the P300 latency clearly reflects the presence of mental retardation, it does not account for differences between patients with this syndrome in their mental ability. Thus, P300 does not appear to have value in assessing the mental abilities of individual Down syndrome individuals.

The results are consistent with the results of the study of Heukrodt et al. (1988) of children who have survived leukemia. Both children with Down syndrome and children who have undergone chemotherapy and the disease process of leukemia show longer latencies than normal controls. However, in the case of children who have recovered from leukemia, P300 latency and cognitive ability were strongly correlated. Similar P300 results were also found by Marsh et al. (in preparation) in relation to patients with very early stage Alzheimer disease. It was found that non-Alzheimer patients and early-stage Alzheimer patients could be easily discriminated by P300 latency, but different levels of mental ability within this narrow range of dementia could not be further discriminated.

Several possible reasons for the failure of P300 latency to account for the mental abilities of the Down syndrome group might be considered. First, P300 latency may not be a sensitive enough measure of mental ability. That is, only relatively large differences in neurocognitive ability are reflected in P300 latency.

Second, the psychometric tests used in this study (primarily the Peabody and Beery) may not themselves represent good measures of mental ability in subjects with Down syndrome. The Beery Developmental Test of Visual-Motor Integration, used to estimate performance mental age for most Down syndrome and all non-Down syndrome subjects, correlates with other measures of performance mental age: 0.50 for first-graders, but only 0.37 for fourth-graders (Beery, 1982). The Peabody Picture Vocabulary Test, used to estimate verbal mental ability, has correlations from 0.04 to 0.88 with the

Weschler Intelligence Scales for Children, Verbal Scale (Dunn & Dunn, 1981). Thus, various instruments for mental ability in children do not necessarily correlate highly, even when purporting to measure the same aspect of ability.

A third reason for the failure of P300 latency to account for the mental and social abilities in the children with Down syndrome may be that P300 latency is predictive of different mental functions in Down syndrome than those assessed by the psychometric measures. Further research regarding predictive validity of P300 latency would be necessary to establish this hypothesis. P300 latency seems to correlate most highly with perceptual recognition speed in normal adults (Brown & Marsh, 1987).

Summary

In conclusion, although the value has been confirmed of P300 latency in the study of cognitive abilities in various childhood disorders, at present, no support exists for the use of P300 latency as an assessment measure for determining the cognitive ability of individual patients with Down syndrome.

References

Beery, K. (1982). *Revised adminstration, scoring, and teaching manual for the development test of visual-motor integration.* Cleveland: Modern Curriculum Press.

Brown, W.S., Marsh, J.T., & LaRue, A. (1982). Event-related potentials in psychiatry: Differentiating depression from dementia in the elderly. *Bulletin of the Los Angeles Neurological Societies, 47*, 91–107.

Brown, W.S., Marsh, J.T., & LaRue, A. (1983). Exponential electrophysiological aging: P300 latency. *Electroencephalography and clinical Neurophysiology, 55* (3), 277–285.

Brown, W.S., & Marsh, J.T. (1987). Unpublished data.

Callner, D.A., & Dustman, R.E. (1975). Developmental trends in the visual, auditory and somatosensory evoked responses of normal and Down syndrome individuals. *Dissertation Abstracts International*, 5249–B.

Callner, D.A., Dustman, R.E., Madsen, J.A., Schenkenberg, T., & Beck, E.C. (1978). Life span changes in the averaged evoked responses of Down's syndrome and non-retarded persons. *American Journal of Mental Deficiency, 82* (4), 398–405.

Connolly, J.A. (1978). Intelligence levels of Down's syndrome children. *American Journal of Mental Deficiency, 83* (2), 193–196.

Courchesne, E. (1977). Event-related brain potentials: Comparison between children and adults. *Science, 197* (4303), 589–592.

Courchesne, E. (1978). Neurophysiological correlates of cognitive development: Changes in long-latency event-related potentials from childhood to adulthood. *Electroencephalography and Clinical Neurophysiology, 45* (4), 468–482.

Crome, L., & Stern, J. (1972). *Pathology of Mental Retardation* (2nd ed.). Edinburgh: Churchill-Livingston.

Duncan-Johnson, C. (1981). P300 latency: A new metric of information processing. *Psychophysiology, 18* (3), 207–215.

Dunn, L., & Dunn, L. (1981). Peabody picture vocabulary test—revised manual for "Form L and M." Minnesota: American Guidance Service.

Galbraith, G. C., Squires, N., Altair, D., & Gliddon, J.B. (1979). Electrophysiological assessments in mentally retarded individuals: From brainstem to cortex. In Henri Begleiter (Ed.), *Evoked brain potentials and behavior* (pp. 229–245). New York: Plenum Publishing Co.

Gliddon, J.B., Busk, J., & Galbraith, G.C. (1975). Visual evoked responses as a function of light intensity in Down's syndrome and nonretarded subjects. *Psychophysiology, 12* (4), 416–422.

Goodin, D.S., Squires, K.C., Henderson, B.H., & Starr, A. (1978). Age-related variations in evoked potentials to auditory stimuli in normal human subjects. *Electroencephalography and Clinical Neurophysiology, 44* (4), 447–458.

Hartley, X.Y. (1986). A summary of recent research into the development of children with Down's syndrome. *Journal of Mental Deficiency Research, 30* (1), 1–14.

Heukrodt, C.M., Powazek, M., Brown, W.S., Kennelly, D., Robinson, H., & Schantz, S. (1988). Evoked response (P300) and neurocognitive status of long-term survivors of childhood leukemia (Vol. 13, No. 2, pp. 223–236).

Kolata, G. (1985). Down syndrome—Alzheimer's linked. *Science, 230*, 1152–1153.

Kutas, M., McCarthy, G., & Donchin, E. (1977). Augmenting mental chronometry: The P300 as a measure of stimulus evaluation time. *Science, 4305*, 792–795.

Lincoln, A.J., Courchesne, E., Kilman, B.A., & Galambos, R. (1985). Neuropsychological correlates of information processing by children with Down syndrome. *American Journal of Mental Deficiency, 89* (4), 403–414.

Marsh, J.T., Brown, W.S., Wolcott, M., Landswerk, J., & Nissenson, A. (1986). Electrophysiological function in hemodialysis and CAPD. *Kidney International, 30*, 957–963.

Marsh, J.T., Schubarth, G., Brown, W.S., Kuhl, D., Reige, W., Strandburg, R., Dorsey, D., & Maltese, A. *PET and P300 relationship in early Alzheimer's disease.* Unpublished manuscript.

McCarthy, G., & Donchin, E.A. (1981). A metric for thought: A comparison of P300 latency and reaction time. *Science, 211* (4477), 77–80.

Morss, J.R. (1983). Cognitive development in the Down syndrome infant: Slow or different? *Brit Journal of Educ. Psychol., 53* (1), 40–47.

Pritchard, W.S. (1981). Psychophysiology of P300. *Psycholog. Bull., 89* (3), 506–540.

Rothenberger, A., & Baschek, V. (1982). P300 in children with different cognitive abilities. In A. Rothenberger (Ed.), *Event-related potentials in children* (pp. 317–323). New York: Elsevier Biomedical Press.

Squires, K.G., Chippendale, T.J., Wrege, K.S., Goodin, D.S., & Starr, A. (1980). Electrophysiological assessment of mental function in aging and dementia. In L.W. Poon (Ed.), *Aging in the 1980's: Psychological issues* (pp. 125–134). Washington, DC: American Psychological Association.

Squires, N.K., Galbraith, G.C., & Aine, C.J. (1979). Event related potential assessment of sensory and cognitive defects in the mentally retarded. In D. Lehmann & E. Callaway (Eds.), *Human Evoked Potentials* (pp. 397–413). New York: Plenum Publishing Co.

Straumanis, J.J., Shagass, C., & Overton, D.A. (1973). Somatosensory evoked

responses in Down syndrome. *Archives of General Psychiatry, 29*(4), 544–549.
Sylvester, P.E. (1983). The hippocampus in Down's syndrome. *Journal of Mental Deficiency Research, 27* (3), 227–236.
Wisniewski, K., Howe, J., Williams, D.G., & Wisniewski, H.M. (1978). Precocious aging and dementia in patients with Down's syndrome. *Biological Psychiatry, 13* (5), 619–627.
Yellin, A.M., Lodwig, A.K., & Jerison, H.T. (1980). Auditory evoked brain potentials as a function of interstimulus interval in adults with Down's syndrome. *Audiology, 19* (3), 255–262.

12
Consonant Phoneme, and Distinctive Feature Error Patterns in Speech

ROBERT W. BORGHI

Introduction

Speech production in the child with Down syndrome appears to be a complex interfacing of disordered systems. Investigation shows the palate of the child with this syndrome to be abnormally short (Austin et al., 1969; Cohen & Cohen, 1971; Gorlin et al., 1976; Shapiro et al., 1967), the tongue excessively large for the oral area (Hohler, 1977, Olbrisch, 1982, Olbrisch, 1985; Wexler et al., 1986), and the musculature to be hypotonic (Smith & Wilson, 1973). Although the palate also appears to be excessively high, investigation confirms that palatal height in these children is within normal limits as compared to other children (Shapiro et al., 1967). Articulatory precision, then, in the child with Down syndrome is thwarted in several dimensions. Both Benda (1949) and Engler (1949) noted early that:

> The oral cavity... is smaller than it should be due to hypoplasia of the maxilla... the net result is a tongue apparently too large for the mouth... [this leads] to clumsiness in the speech production because of the difficulty involved in accurate use of the tongue (Zisk & Bialer, 1967, p. 235).

The question of inadequate articulatory precision leading to poor intelligibility has frustrated parents and therapists. To improve tongue control, and thus articulation, as well as both swallowing and appearance, increasing attention has been given to surgical modification of the tip of the tongue (Hohler, 1977; Olbrisch, 1985; Rozner, 1983), thereby decreasing tongue length for improved intraoral control. Although the data are scanty, some improvement in articulation (intelligibility) and swallowing has been reported (Hohler, 1977; Rozner, 1983; Wexler et al., 1986). This information has come principally from parent reports, not from formal study. Although surgical intervention is drastic and certainly irreversible, a great many parents in our test population expressed interest in taking early steps that would improve the life-long communication, swallowing, and facial appearance of their children.

The literature expounding improvement is not clear as to those sounds or lingual movements that have been improved by surgically modifying tongue length. Before consideration of permanent changes in muscle tissue, some attention must be directed toward exploring the articulatory error pattern of these children, not only to identify allophonic variation and phoneme substitution, but also to delineate the error pattern of their distinctive features. One approach to the problem is to examine the articulatory movements through an assessment format that includes distinctive features of each consonant phoneme. With these needs in mind, the Fisher-Logemann Test of Articulation Competence was selected as one of the test instruments in evaluating the speech production of the children in a Down syndrome program.

Patient Population

One-hundred-ninety children with Down syndrome from 6 months to 19 years of age were evaluated by an interdisciplinary team over an 18-month period. Each child was evaluated for approximately two days. The speech evaluation was scheduled for a one-hour period. Each child was accompanied by a parent or guardian during the test period.

Fifty subjects successfully completed the Fisher-Logemann Test and were included in this study. The test group of 50 subjects comprised 25 males and 25 females ranging in age from 5.0 to 19.1 years. The median age was 9.2 years.

To compare performance, the group was divided into three age categories: Category I, 5.0–7.11 years; Category II, 8.0–11.9 years; and Category III, 12.0–19.1 years.

Category I comprised 15 subjects: 10 males, 5 females; the median age was 5.10 years. Category II comprised 21 subjects: 10 males, 11 females; the median age was 9.2 years. Category III comprised 14 subjects: 5 males, 9 females. The median age was 14.8 years.

Procedures and Methods

Testing was conducted in a quiet room with little ambient noise. Each child was accompanied by a parent or guardian who remained in the test area during evaluation.

Each child was administered the Fisher-Logemann Test of Articulation Competence. Each test session was tape-recorded on a Sony M19Z cassette recorder and reviewed for the accuracy of the phonetic transcriptions.

The test was conducted as per test protocol whenever possible. When a subject could not remember the name of a stimuli object or did not know the name, it was provided. The test authors stipulate that, "Saying the word for the subject to imitate should be avoided, *except* when the patient is known to have a severe word-finding problem" (Fisher & Logemann, 1971, p. 13).

Each error response was recorded in the appropriate designated cell on the test record form. Although the individual allophonic modification and phoneme substitutions were recorded for therapy planning and therapy guidance, the major thrust of the testing was to determine the focus of major error patterns of the consonant phonemes, and the error patterns of those distinctive features that are most affected by the structural, muscular, and neurological deficits in the oral area of children with Down syndrome. A second focus was to determine the error patterns that seem to be the most resistant to change. For convenience and clarity, each cell used on the test record form was assigned a number in consecutive order. Since only consonant phonemes were the focus there were 65 cells.

In data collection for consonant phonemes, each error in each vocalic position was counted as a single error. The collective data for each phoneme was the total number of errors recorded.

The data collected for the distinctive feature error pattern was the error count in each cognate pair and each single consonant. Data analysis revealed no additional information was gained by separating the phoneme cognates and including the voicing feature.

A percentage of error was struck after summing each group of cells. For each consonant phoneme in each category a final percentage of errors was

TABLE 12.1. Percentage of error of consonant phonemes.

Cell	Consonant phoneme	Category I	Category II	Category III
1–3	p	0.02	0.06	0.02
4–6	b	0.20	0.05	0.12
7–8	m	0.27	0.05	0.21
9–11	w	0.09	0.02	0.05
12–14	f	0.29	0.17	0.12
15–17	v	0.62[8]	0.48[7]	0.38[6]
18–20	θ	0.76[2]	0.60[6]	0.45[3]
21–23	ð	0.71[3]	0.63[4]	0.62[1]
24–26	t	0.31	0.11	0.12
27–29	d	0.33	0.15	0.12
30–32	l	0.33	0.16	0.14
33–35	n	0.31	0.09	0.12
36–38	s	0.67[6]	0.48[8]	0.45[4]
39–41	z	0.93[1]	0.63[2]	0.50[2]
42–44	ʃ	0.71[4]	0.68[1]	0.38[5]
45–47	tʃ	0.71[5]	0.62[5]	0.26
48–50	dʒ	0.62[7]	0.63[3]	0.33[7]
51–52	j	0.40	0.26	0.29[8]
53–55	r	0.40	0.22	0.24
56–58	k	0.29	0.13	0.02
59–61	g	0.33	0.16	0.17
62–63	ŋ	0.37	0.31	0.32
64–65	h	0.13	0.09	0.07

Category I = 5.0–7.11 yrs; Category II = 8.0–11.9 yrs; Category III = 12.0–19.1 yrs; 1–8 ranked order of magnitude of error.

calculated. The same procedure was followed to calculate a final percentage of error for the distinctive feature analysis.

The data was rank-ordered to identify those consonant phonemes and distinctive features that showed the highest error patterns in each category. Table 12.1 delineates, in percentage form, the total error count for each consonant phoneme. The data are presented by age category.

The distinctive feature data are presented in Table 12.2. The consonant cognates are grouped together with no effort to include the voicing feature.

Results

The child with Down syndrome appears to have continuing articulation/intelligibility difficulties throughout life. The essential focus of this study was to determine which consonant phonemes were the most error-prone and resistant to change, and which distinctive features of the articulate phonemes share this resistance. Table 12.1 shows the percentage of error for each phoneme tested for the three age-group categories. Careful examination of

TABLE 12.2. Percentage of error of distinctive features of consonant phonemes.

Cell	Consonant phonemes	Distinctive features	Category I	Category II	Category III
1–6	p,b	Bilabial stop	0.22	0.05	0.07
7–8	w	Bilabial glide	0.27	0.05	0.21
9–11	m	Bilabial nasal	0.09	0.02	0.05
12–17	f,v	Labio-dental fricative	0.45[5]	0.32[5]	0.25
18–23	θ,ð	Tip-dental fricative	0.73[2]	0.62[3]	0.54[1]
24–29	t,d	Tip-alveolar stop	0.32	0.13	0.12
30–32	l	Tip-alveolar lateral	0.33	0.16	0.14
33–35	n	Tip-alveolar nasal	0.31	0.09	0.12
36–41	s,z	Blade-alveolar fricative	0.80[1]	0.55[4]	0.48[2]
42–44	ʃ	Blade-prepalatal fricative	0.71[3]	0.68[1]	0.38[3]
45–50	tʃ,dʒ	Blade-prepalatal affricate	0.67[4]	0.63[2]	0.30
51–52	j	Front palatal glide	0.40	0.26	0.29
53–55	r	Central palatal glide	0.40	0.22	0.38[4]
56–61	k,g	Back velar stop	0.31	0.14	0.09
62–63	ŋ	Back velar nasal	0.37	0.31	0.32[5]
64–65	h	Glottal fricative	0.13	0.09	0.07

[1-5]Ranked order of magnitude of error.

Category I shows that the consonant phonemes (listed in descending order: /z/,/θ/,/ð/,/ʃ/,/tʃ/,/ s/,/dʒ/, and /v/ are the most difficult sounds to articulate for this age group. These phonemes, however, are also the most difficult for age Categories II and III. The order of difficulty is different, but these phonemes continue to be difficult.

A further examination of Table 12.1 shows a reduction in percentage of error as age increases. Whether this is a product of age or training can only be conjectured, but it is worth noting that some phonemes are very resistant to change. The /ð/,/z/,/θ/,/s/, and /ʃ/ are notable in this regard. Tongue control is a continuing problem, although some diminishment in percentage of error is seen as the child moves to adolescence.

A second way to examine articulation is to examine the distinctive features that combine to produce the phoneme. Table 12.2 delineates in percentages the error pattern of the manner of formation and place of articulation. Relying on manner and place (eliminating the voicing feature), the distinctive features can be studied. The cells holding the phoneme cognates or single phoneme with highest error percentage in Category I are the fricative/affricates in combination with the features of blade/alveolar, tip/dental, blade/prepalatal, and labio/dental. Identical error patterns are found in Category II subjects, although the order of magnitude is altered. In Category III the pattern is carried forward, but with some modification. The /f/ and /v/ phonemes are found at a slightly lower level of severity, but the remaining distinctive features remain the same. There is also an increase in degree of difficulty for the /1/ (glide, central palatal), and /ŋ/ (nasal, back velar). Other than continuing difficulties in feature control, the increase in difficulty for the /1/ and /ŋ/ are puzzling, in that they are not high in error percentage in Categories I and II.

Improvement in tongue control by whatever means appears to be a critical element in improving articulation in the child with Down syndrome. Although research does little to verify it, clinical experience seems to show that bringing the articulators under control early in the child's life promotes a better articulatory picture and a more intelligible child.

Summary

Fifty children with Down syndrome between the ages of 5 and 19 years were divided by age into three categories. Category I included children between the ages of 5 and 7.11 years, Category II 8.0 and 11.9 years, and Category III children from 12.0 to 19.1 years old. Each group was given the Fisher-Logemann Test of Articulation Competence in random order. The focus of the data compilation was to determine the major error patterns of consonant articulation and the error patterns of the distinctive features that interact to produce these phonemes.

Data analysis indicates that seven phonemes appear to be most error-prone and resistant to change. These phonemes, in descending rank order, are /z/, /θ/,/ð/,/ʃ/,/tʃ/,/dʒ/, and /v/.

The distinctive features found to be the most error-prone are the fricative/affricates, combined with the features of blade/alveolar, tip/dental, blade/prepalatal, and labio/dental. The anterior tongue, as expected, plays a major role in continuing faulty articulation in children with Down syndrome.

References

Austin, J.H., Pregar, L., Siris, E., & Taybi, H. (1969). Short hard palate in newborn, roentgen sign of Mongolism. *Radiology, 92*, 775–776.

Benda, C.E. (1949). *Mongolism and cretinism.* New York: Grune and Stratton Publishing.

Cohen, M.M.,& Cohen, M.M. (1971). The oral manifestations of trisomy G_1 (Down syndrome). *Birth defects: Original article series, III* (7), 241–251.

Engler, M. (1949). *Mongolism.* Bristol, England: John Wright.

Fisher, H.B., & Logemann, J.A. (1971). *The Fisher-Logemann test of articulation competence.* Boston: Houghton Mifflin.

Gorlin, R.J., Pindborg, J.J., & Cohen, M.M. (1976). *Syndromes of the head and neck.* New York: McGraw-Hill.

Hohler, H. (1977). Changes in facial expression as a result of plastic surgery in Mongoloid children. *Aesthetic Plas Sur, 1*, 250–253.

Lemperle, G., & Radu, D. (1980). Facial plastic surgery in children with Down's syndrome. *Plas and Reconstr. Surg, 66*, 337–342.

Olbrisch, R.R. (1982). Plastic surgical management of children with Down's syndrome: Indications and results. *Brit Journal of Plas Surg, 35*, 195–200.

Olbrisch, R.R. (1985). Plastic and aesthetic surgery on children with Down's syndrome. *Aesthetic Plastic Surgery, 9*, 241–248.

Rozner, L. (1983). Facial plastic surgery for Down's syndrome. *Lancet, 11* (1:8337), 1320–1323.

Shapiro, B.L., Gorlin, R.J., Redman, R.S., & Brush, H.H. (1967). The palate and Down's syndrome. *New England Journal of Medicine, 276*, 1460–1463.

Smith, D., & Wilson, A. (1973). *The child with Down's syndrome (Mongolism): Causes, characteristics, and acceptance.* Philadelphia: W.B. Saunders.

Wexler, M.R., Peled, I.J., Rand, Y., Mintzker, Y., & Feverstein, R. (1986). Rehabilitation of the face in patients with Down's syndrome. *Plas and Reconstr Surg, 77* (3), 383–391.

Zisk, P.K., & Bialer, I. (1967). Speech and language problems in Mongolism: A review of the literature. *J of Speech and Hear Disorders, 32* (3), 228–241.

13
Language Development and Intervention

LAURA F. MEYERS

Introduction

Children with Down syndrome usually have particular difficulties with, and delays in, language development (Miller, 1987, 1988). They often do not acquire words until their second year, and may not combine words until their third or fourth year. As they reach the age when children without handicaps begin to use grammatical sentences, they typically continue to convey complex meanings through simple sequences of words in telegraphic speech. Many fail to learn the rules they need to form grammatically correct sentences. Even when children with Down syndrome seem to have mastered some language skill, they will often use their new vocabulary or language structure inconsistently, while continuing to use the kinds of words and structure characteristic of much younger children.

There are many causes for language delay in children with Down syndrome, affecting development of both comprehension and production of language. These include:

1. a greater frequency of otitis media, serous infections, and fluid in the middle ear (Berko-Gleason, 1983; Bess, 1983), a greater incidence of mild to moderate hearing loss, structural differences in the middle ear and ear canal, and an increased build up of wax in the ear canal. All of these problems can impair hearing acuity, resulting in delayed and deviant development of *comprehension* of language (Chapter 3, this volume; Downs, 1981; Klein, et al., 1984)
2. delayed and/or deviant motor development, with prevalent hypotonia, which can cause problems with control of the tongue, lips, and breathstream for speech. These problems can result in delayed and deviant *articulation*, as well as deviant and delayed development of *production* of language (Miller, 1987, 1988)
3. moderate to severe retardation in cognitive development that may make it difficult to learn to understand the meaning of the complex, rapid, auditory stream of speech (Marcell & Armstrong, 1982; Morss, 1983; Silverstein et al., 1982; Smart et al., 1982)

Results of Language Assessment of Children with Down Syndrome

What Is Language?

In order to understand the results of language assessments reported here and in the literature, it is useful to first review the system of language as a whole. Language is a formal system of rules that children and adults use to convey meaning through sound. The function of language is to communicate to another person an intended meaning through sound. When children have constructed an internal set of language rules, or grammar, they can understand sentences that they have never before heard and produce sentences that they have never before said.

Language has a number of components. *The components of language are:*

Vocabulary. Does the child have the *number* of words expected for her/his age? Does the child know the *different kinds of words* needed to construct sentences, including names of objects and people (*nouns:* ball, Dad), names of actions (*verbs:* eat, sleep), words about locations (*prepositions:* into, under), descriptive words (*adjectives:* big, green), *articles* (the, a), time words (*adverbs:* tomorrow).

Phonetics. This area covers how well *sound* is used in understanding and speaking. Can the child *intentionally articulate* the sounds needed to communicate? Can the child *discriminate* the sounds of English?

Phonology. This area covers how well the child has mastered the *meaningful sounds* of language. Does the child know which sounds make a *meaning difference* in the language? Does the child know that *b*at, *c*at, *p*at, *h*at, *f*at, *s*at, *m*at, and *r*at all mean something different, so that substitution of one sound for another makes a difference in meaning in the language?

Morphology. Children know the morphology of their language when they know the rules for *adding markets to nouns and verbs* to add the meaning of plural, time etc. Does the child know how to form *regular plurals*, adding -*s*(cat → cat*s*), or how to form *irregular plurals* (child → child*ren*, wom*a*n → wom*e*n)? Does the child know how to form *regular past tenses*, by adding -*ed* (stop → stopp*ed*), or how to form *irregular past tenses* (go → *went*, eat → *ate*)?

Syntax. Syntactic rules of language let the child construct sentences with correct *order of words*. Does the child know how to *sequence words* into developmentally appropriate sentences? (Example. "I can see the dog" is syntactically correct, "See the can I dog" is not.) Does the child know that the *word order is different* for statements and questions ("I can see the dog" → "Can I see the dog?")

Semantics and Pragmatics. Rules governing how to use language to convey and understand *meaning*, and to *carry on a conversation* with another person are rules of semantics and pragmatics. Does the child know how to spontaneously convey personal meaning, i.e., to get a listener to understand what (s)he is talking about? Does the child know how to begin and maintain a conversation?

When a child with Down syndrome is evaluated for language functioning, each component should be assessed. In speech and language intervention, a good program will include goals and methods to improve functioning in all of these components. Children's grammars change as they develop. What is an appropriate utterance for a two year old is ungrammatical for a four-year-old.

When children are learning *written* language, the same areas of language functioning should be addressed. Child need to learn written vocabulary; they need learn to use text to mark nouns and verbs for number and time; they need to learn to sequence words correctly in writing; and they need to use written language to convey meaning. In addition, they need to learn to associate letters with the sounds of language, and with the meanings associated with those sounds.

What Are the Characteristics of Language Development in Children with Down Syndrome?

In this section, language development in children with Down syndrome will be described. First, results of language assessments of the child population with Down syndrome described in Chapter 1 will be presented. Then the characteristics of infants, toddlers, preschoolers, and school-aged children will be described using this information as well as findings from previous research reports.

Methods and Patient Population. A total of 110 children with Down syndrome received full language assessments at the City of Hope during the project period (1985–88). Standardized language tests were given. Children under 91 months (7.6 years) chronological age were given the Bzoch-League Receptive-Expressive Language Scale (REEL) and the Sequenced Inventory of Communication Development (SICD). Children over 91 months were given the Illinois Test of Psycholinguistic Abilities (ITPA) and the Peabody Picture Vocabulary Test (PPVT). In addition, all children were videotaped in spontaneous interactions with their caretakers, the researcher, and appropriate toys and objects. The tapes were analyzed to determine the spontaneous expressive language level of the children. The results of the standardized testing are presented in Table 13.1.

Figure 13.1 presents graphically two patterns of development that were found during the language assessment that are of considerable concern. First, there is a downturn in development at 19–24 months, in both comprehension and production. This is due to lack of acquisition of first words and word

TABLE 13.1. Results of standardized testing.[a]

Age months (N)	Comprehension Mean ls	76+ ls(%)	Range of ls	75− ls(%)	Range of ls	Production Mean ls	76+ ls(%)	Range of ls	75− ls(%)	Range of ls
0–6 (7)	66	43	100	57	33	54	14	100	86	17–66
7–12 (10)	75	40	76–82	60	60–75	71	30	76–83	70	60–75
13–18 (12)	73	58	79–94	42	38–69	67	42	79–94	58	38–73
19–24 (11)	61	36	78–81	64	53–73	63	36	81–86	64	48–74
25–30 (9)	72	55	79–114	45	26–71	68	45	76–100	55	26–71
31–40 (12)	64	25	78–88	75	42–71	62	17	78–81	83	38–70
41–60 (15)	51	13	77–86	87	23–64	51	7	77	93	23–71
61–90 (14)	47	0		100	15–71	42	0		100	10–72
91–144 (12)	41	0		100	31–50	39	0		100	33–56
145–228 (8)	38	0		100	15–53	34	0		100	13–60
Total (110)	59					55				

[a] REEL and SICD were used with children with chronological ages less than 91 mos. (7.6 yrs); PPVT and ITPA were used with children over 91 mos. For each age group, for both comprehension and production of language, mean language score(ls) is provided, % of children performing above and below 75%, along with the range of language scores within each age group.

combinations. Second, after 30 months, there is a progressive continuing decline in both comprehension and production abilities. This is due to deficiencies in acquisition of the syntactic and morphological language structures used to form sentences.

Results of analysis of the videotaped language interactions clearly demonstrated the same delays as were found in the standardized testing. The results

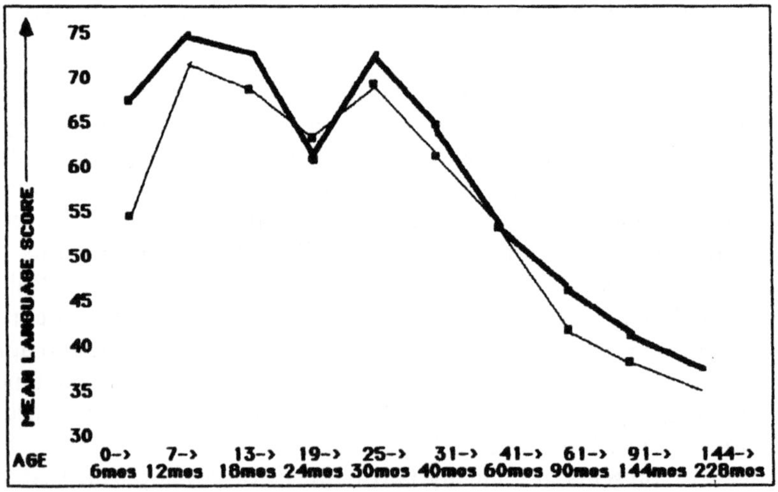

FIGURE 13.1. Mean language scores on standardized tests: Comprehension (thick line) and production (thin line) for each age group.

TABLE 13.2. Results of analysis of videotaped language interactions.[a]

Chronological age (Mos.)	Best Productive Utterance Type			
	Voc/Bab/Jar	Words	Word comb	Sentences
0–6	100	0	0	0
7–12	100	0	0	0
13–18	83	17	0	0
19–24	55	36	9	0
25–30	11	67	22	0
31–40	16	34	50	0
41–60	0	48	40	12
61–90	8	21	21	50
91–144	8	17	8	67
144+	0	0	25	75

[a]For each age group, the percent of subjects with best productive utterance within each utterance type was recorded. The lowest productive utterance type was vocalization, babbling or jargon, followed by single words, word combinations, and grammatical sentences.

are shown in Table 13.2, which documents the best productive utterance type occurring during the taped language samples.

In children without handicaps, first words typically appear by 10–12 months. By 19–21 months children without handicaps usually have between 20–50 words (Miller & Chapman, 1987). Of the children with Down syndrome, no child had any words before 12 months, and at 12–18 months only 17% of the toddlers with Down syndrome uttered any words during the videotaped interaction. It was not until age 25–30 months that a majority of the children with Down syndrome used words.

The use of word combinations was also considerably delayed. Children without handicaps combine words by 19 months (Miller, 1981). For half of the children with Down syndrome, it was not until 31–40 months that they formed any word combinations.

In children without handicaps, beginning sentences appear between 31 and 34 months (Miller, 1981). In the subject population with Down syndrome, no child had sentences until 41–60 months. At 61–90 months only 50% of the children with Down syndrome uttered any sentences during the videotaped interaction; the other children still used single words, word combinations, and even vocalizations.

Characteristics of Language Development in Children with Down Syndrome

During infancy the main areas of language development are: (a) phonetics and phonology (development of the sound system, in particular, learning to pay attention to and to produce sounds), and (b) semantics and pragmatics (learning to carry on a "conversation," taking turns making sounds, and beginning to understand that speech sounds (words) have meaning). Many babies with Down syndrome are unusually quiet. They are often described as "good babies" because they do not fuss and make noise. Parents notice that they are not as aware of sound in their environment as other children. On testing, three characteristics stand out. First, these children may not search out people while they are talking in order to watch their mouths to see how sounds are made as much as babies without handicaps do. Second, they tend not to babble a lot of different sounds, repeating them over and over, the way babies without handicaps do. Some people feel that babbling leads to language development and that it is good for babies to babble, because it helps them begin to say words. Third, babies with Down syndrome often need to be encouraged to interact with their caregivers, taking their turn during sound-play games. The caregivers have to work extra hard to get these interactions going; once the games are begun their babies enjoy playing social games, such as peek-a-boo, as much as babies without handicaps do.

The delay in acquisition of first words by toddlers, documented with the project children, has also been found by other researchers (Fowler, 1988; Miller, 1988; Stoel-Gammon, 1980). One researcher reported on a group of children with this syndrome who were enrolled in an excellent language intervention project from birth. The children with Down syndrome in that project acquired the first words at 21 months, 7 months after the non-Down control group. Rate and use of meaningful words for the 10 months following the appearance of the first words was even more delayed. At 31 months, only 10% of utterances of the children with Down syndrome were judged to be attempts at real words, while for the normal control group, 100% of their vocalizations were judged as meaningful at 24 months, 10 months after their first words had appeared (Stoel-Gammon, 1980).

The most striking fact about the language development of the project preschoolers and school-aged children was that many of them did not acquire the small function words and morphological markets that are used to form sentences, similarly to the children studied by other researchers (Rempel, 1974; Strominger et al., 1984). Their semantics and pragmatics were at a much higher level than their morphology and syntax. They often used sequences of single words or word combinations to convey complex meanings. Many of the older children would utter a grammatical sentence one moment, and then continue the same conversation using multiword or single word utterances (for example: "I like Cathy. Her nice. Pretty.") Some of the teenagers could speak in grammatical sentences, but they used very simple sentences with language structure more characteristic of a three to four year old, although the content was more sophisticated. Their articulation was often quite poor, and they showed or said that they felt embarrassed and frustrated when asked to repeat. They preferred to drop the topic, rather than trying to make themselves understood. Others among the older children would keep trying to make their point, but they had very few ways to make their messages clear. These higher functioning children would make the same errors in their speech that three- to four-year-old children without handicaps do for example, overgeneralizing the past tense rule, saying things like "she goed" or "he thinked." Analysis of the videotaped interactions showed that no child consistently used sentence structure correctly, at any age level.

Language Intervention

Suggested language interventions for infants and children with Down syndrome are presented here and in Table 13.3. For infants with Down syndrome, language intervention should promote development of attention to sound, producing sounds, and linking sound to meaning. Hearing should be evaluated as early as possible (See chapter 2, this volume), and should be reevaluated during the first three years any time that loss is suspected (due to ear

TABLE 13.3. Language interventions.

Infants

Language development goals: paying attention to sound and to how sounds are made; taking turns in sound-play games; babbling different sounds; beginning to understand that words (sounds) have meaning; producing first words.

Interventions: Evaluate hearing often; set up a routine of sound-play games (caretakers repeat same routine daily, exaggerate sounds and facial expressions, give the infant time to take a turn by smiling, squirming, squealing or vocalizing), peek-a-boo, patty-cake, favorite songs; looking at picture books and playing with toys using the same language daily; infant stimulation program to learn from professionals and other parents about ways to encourage baby's language development.

Toddlers and Preschoolers

Language development goals: Understanding words for people, objects and actions; producing first words, learning to use words to talk about people, objects and actions; producing first word combinations; learning how to use language to communicate with another person.

Interventions: Continuing to repeat play and daily living routines at home, using similar language on a daily basis; augmenting the speech signal with toys, objects, actions, sign language, picture books, and computer-generated speech output and monitor graphics; preschool (nonhandicapped) with good peer language models; preschool (special) with enriched language classroom.

School-Aged Children

Language development goals: Learning to understand and produce language structure; learning the morphology of language (function words such as *do, is, not, the* and markers such as plural, past tense, and possessives); learning higher level vocabulary; learning to use written language to learn about spoken language structure; learning how to choose a topic and develop it; learning how to use language in conversations with other people.

Interventions: Give teachers a list of vocabulary words and sentence types that the child uses (with a pronunciation guide); learn about the development of language structure so that new structure can be introduced at the correct developmental age; acknowledge the content of what the child says, then provide the correct language structure to express the message; write on computers with speech output to help make the sound-meaning link; give the child guidance beforehand about how best to convey a message to another person; observe the classroom and generalize what is being learned there to the home and other situations.

infections, lack of attention to sound, etc.). As the infant matures, more and more thorough hearing evaluation becomes possible. It is particularly important to determine that the infant has hearing adequate for all the sounds of speech. Babies will enjoy sound play the most if they can predict the routines that the caregivers use each day. Caregivers interacting with babies naturally exaggerate sounds and intonation patterns. Babies enjoy these unusual sounds and watch to see how they are made. Calling attention to the mouth, by making funny sounds with the lips, sticking the tongue out, and putting the babies' fingers on the mouth, helps babies find out how the sounds are made. It is very easy, out of concern for the baby, to try too hard to get the baby to make sounds. It is important that caregivers pause in their sound-making to let the babies take their turn. At first, the babies may take their turn by smiling, squirming or dancing up and down with their hands and feet. This should be acknowledged and accepted. Any sound the baby makes should be met with praise and smiles. Babies like it when caretakers repeat their sounds, making them important. All babies need regular time-outs when they can turn away from the interaction with their caretakers. This should be allowed and encouraged, and when the babies spontaneously return to the interaction, they should be welcomed back with quiet encouragement (Stern, 1977).

It is important, beginning in the middle of the first year, to use toys, pictures, and objects to help the babies link speech sounds (words) with meaning. Playing with interesting toys, picture books, and objects on a daily basis, at a predictable time, repeating the same language each day, helps all developing babies begin to guess which speech sounds are linked with which toys and events. As they begin to understand words, they will spontaneously try to say them. Toys, picture books, objects, and actions augment the child's language environment, i.e., they provide nonverbal cues to the meaning of the speech sounds. All children need these augmentative cues to begin to learn language. Another way to augment speech during the second and third year is to introduce a small sign language vocabulary into the children's established play and daily living routines. For children with Down syndrome who have problems analyzing and producing speech sounds, signs are an excellent way to help them actively participate in early language activities. First words in speech are learned, forgotten, and learned again (the way children without handicaps learn). Signs often remain stable. Signs help children communicate the meanings of the spoken words they represent. Research has found that augmenting spoken language with visual forms of communication helps children learn language and has beneficial effects on their behavior (Silverman, 1980).

Another way to help toddlers and preschoolers begin to understand and produce words is to augment the play and language sessions with computer-generated synthesized speech output linked with computer monitor graphics (Meyers, 1986, 1987, 1988, 1990). It is important that the software put the speech output and graphics completely under the control of the children, rather than simply using them to instruct the children. Children need to control the speech output and graphics in order to benefit from their advantages as tools that they can use to learn to understand and produce language. Speech output is a wonderful tool to use to begin to understand the sound patterns of words and language structure, because it can occur at a slower rate than conversational human speech, with each segment of the word completely specified in the speech signal. Human speech is characterized by its rapid rate (2.9–5 syllables per second, each syllable having at least two segments; Pickett, 1980). In human speech, segments are often eliminated entirely, or are missing some information as they are assimilated to the articulation of preceding or following segments. Each time a word is said, by the same or different speakers, the acoustic signal changes. Computer-generated speech output lets children repeat the same slow speech signal for a word as many times they need to hear it. Children with Down syndrome immediately recognize speech output as a powerful tool.

Speech output can also help children with Down syndrome produce language. It can function as a voice to immediately let them enter a conversation, using the auditory-vocal modalities of language. As they experience the powerful function of language, to communicate to another speaker/hearer an intended message through sound, they become more motivated to try to produce the words on their own. They notice the differences between their own articulation of a word and that of the speech output. They use the speech output to practice their words, gradually bringing their own productions closer to the more correct signal of the speech output. For instance, one 20 month old toddler with Down syndrome activated the computer to hear the word *more*. He immediately said, "or" in his own speech. Then, he activated the speech output again, repeating "bor." He had figured out that the word began with some way of putting the lips together. Finally, he activated the speech output again, said, "more," and applauded himself. He had used the speech output to figure out that the word began with the nasal *m*.

When computer-generated speech output is linked to computer monitor graphics under the child's control, the visual signal of the monitor graphics helps the child remember what word was produced in the speech output. Since the visual abilities of toddlers with Down syndrome are usually at a higher level than their auditory skills, these children demonstrate their delight at being able to produce a picture on a computer monitor screen that they understand.

To test for the effectiveness of computer-enhanced language interventions using speech output and computer monitor graphics, a research project funded by the National Institutes of Health was carried out (Meyers, 1988). In the NIH study, toddlers and preschoolers with Down syndrome were enrolled in computer-enhanced and standard language interventions (without the computer present). They played with age-appropriate toys and used the computer, sign language and speech to talk about their play. The effectiveness of the different types of language intervention in promoting vocabulary learning and use, by each subject, were compared. Data analysis of the results showed that the toddlers with Down syndrome learned and used language best when they controlled monitor graphics or both speech output and monitor graphics.

With school-aged children with Down syndrome, the focus of language intervention should be on the development of language structure. In the acoustic signal for speech, the grammatical markers that tie words together into sentences are all characterized by short duration, reduced stress, and low volume. These include words such as *do, is, will, not the, a, her*, and *he*. Other grammatical markers are added to nouns and verbs to add an additional meaning, such as *-s* (plural, as in car*s*), *-ed* (past tense, as in stopp*ed*), *-'s* (possessive, as in John'*s*) *n't* (negative as in is*n't*) and *-est* (superlative, as in bigg*est*). As mentioned earlier in this chapter, children with Down syndrome have an increased incidence of hearing problems, and poorer auditory memory than other children. It is probable that they are not aware that these short grammatical markers are even present in the speech addressed to them. They need intervention that makes language structure more salient.

One way to enhance, or augment, the speech signal is to use writing (Meyers, 1986, 1987, 1988, in press). All of the grammatical markers are obvious in text, and the visual signal of text on a page remains stable, rather than appearing and disappearing at a rapid rate and changing constantly the way the speech signal does. Another research study, funded by the Easter Seal Research Foundation, was carried out with school-aged children with Down syndrome to test the effectiveness of an intervention during which the children wrote about the topics of their choice on a computer that "said" the letters, words and sentences in speech output as they wrote. During the project period, their writing was collected into a 30-page book that they took home at the end of their participation in the study. The researchers encouraged the children to express their thoughts about the topics of their choice and then provided the children with the language structure they needed to express their thoughts in grammatical sentences. The speech output linked the visual text that they created on the monitor screen with the auditory-vocal signal of speech (Meyers, 1988). The hypothesis was that writing on computers with speech output would help the children learn spoken language structure.

Preliminary data analysis confirmed the hypothesis. The children used more age-appropriate grammatical utterances in their spontaneous speech during and after their sessions writing on the computer with speech output than during sessions writing on the computer without speech output or during the standard intervention. Observational and anecdotal evidence indicated a definite improvement in the children's spoken language performance, both receptive and expressive, at home and in school. It was reported that the children's interest in and use of reading and writing skills at home and in school increased during their work on the project.

Summary

Children with Down syndrome have particular difficulties and delays in language development. Even when they seem to have mastered some language skills, they often fail to form grammatically correct sentences, frequently use new vocabulary or language structure inconsistently, and continue to use words and structure characteristic of much younger children. Specific language interventions that link the auditory signal of speech with visual signals such as signs, computer monitor graphics and text are the most likely to help children with Down syndrome make progress learning language.

References

Berko-Gleason, J. (1983). Otitis media and language development. In C. Bluestone et al. (Eds.), Workshop on effects of otitis media on the child, *Pediatrics, 71*(4), 644–645.

Bess, F. (1983). Hearing associated with middle ear effusion. In C. Bluestone et al., Workshop on effects of otitis media on the child, *Pediatrics, 71* (4), 640–641.

Brickner, D. (1972). Imitative sign training as a facilitator of work-object association with low functioning children. *American Journal of Mental Deficiency, 76*, 506–516.

Downs, M. (1980). The hearing of Down's individuals, M. Downs. *Seminars in Speech, Language, and Hearing, 1* (1), 25–38.

Fowler, A. (1988). Determinations of rate of language growth in children with Down syndrome. In L. Nadel (Ed.), *Psychobiology of Down syndrome* (pp. 217–246). Boston: MIT Press.

Klein, J., Teele, D., Mannos, R., Menyuk, P., & Rosner, B. (1984). Otitis media with effusion during the first three years of life and development of speech and language. In Lim, Bluestone, Klein, & Nelson, (Eds.), *Recent advances in otitis media with effusion.* New York: B. Decker, Inc.

Leifer, J.S., & Lewis, M. (1984). Acquisition of conversational response skills by young Down syndrome and non-retarded young children. *American Journal of Mental Deficiency, 88*(6), 610–618.

Marcell, M., & Armstrong, V. (1982). Auditory and visual sequential memory of Down syndrome and non-retarded children. *American Journal of Mental Deficiency, 87* (1), 86–95.

Meyers, L. (1984a). Unique contribution of microcomputers to language intervention with handicapped children. In L. Meyers (Ed.), *Augmenting language skills with microcomputers, seminars in speech and language, 5* (1), 23–34.

Meyers, L. (1984b). Use of microprocessors to imitate language in young nonoral children. In W. Perkins (Ed.), *Current therapy of communication disorders: Language handicaps in children.* New York: Thieme-Stratton.

Meyers, L. (1986). Teaching language. *Exceptional Parent Magazine, 16* (7), 20–23.

Meyers, L. (1987). Bypassing the prerequisites: The computer as a language scaffold. *Closing the gap, 5* (6), 19–20.

Meyers, L. (1988). Using computers to teach children with Down syndrome spoken and written language skills. In L. Nadel (Ed.), *Psychobiology of Down syndrome* (pp. 247–265). Boston: MIT Press.

Meyers, L. (1990). *The language machine.* Boston: College Hill Press.

Miller, J. (1981). *Assessing language production in children.* Baltimore: University Park Press.

Miller, J. (1987). Language and communication characteristics of children with Down syndrome. In S. Pueschel et al. (Eds.), *New perspectives on Down syndrome.* Baltimore: PH Brookes Publishing Co.

Miller, J. (1988). Developmental asynchrony of language development in children with Down syndrome. In L. Nadel (Ed.), *Psychobiology of Down syndrome* (pp. 167–198). Boston: MIT Press.

Miller, J., & Chapman, R. (1981). The relation between age and mean length of utterance in morphemes. *J Sp and Hear Res, 24,* 154–161.

Morss, J. (1983). Cognitive development in the Down's syndrome infant: Slow or different? *Brit J Educ Psych, 53,* 40–47.

O'Connor, N., & Hermelin, B. (1978). *Seeing and hearing and space and time.* London, U.K.: Academic Press.

Pickett, J. (1980). *The sounds of speech communication.* Baltimore: University Park Press.

Rempel, E. (1974). Psycholinguistic abilities of Down's syndrome children. *Proceedings of the Annual Meeting of the AAMD,* Toronto, Canada.

Silverman, F. (1980). *Communication for the speechless.* New Jersey: Prentice-Hall.

Silverstein, A., Legutki, G., Friedman, S., & Takayama, D. (1982). Performance of Down syndrome individuals on the Stanford-Binet intelligence scale. *American Journal of Mental Deficiency, 86* (5), 548–551.

Smart, F., O'Grady, M., & Das, J. (1982). Cognitive processing by subgroups of moderately mentally retarded children. *American Journal of Mental Deficiency, 86* (5), 465–472.

Stark, J., Rosenbaum, R.L., Schwartz, D., & Wisan, A. (1973). The non-verbal child: Some clinical guidelines. *JSHD, 38* (1), 59–71.

Stern, D. (1977). *The first relationship: Infant and mother.* Cambridge, MA: Harvard University Press.

Stoel-Gammon, C. (1980). Speech development in infants and children with Down's syndrome. In J. Darby, Jr. (Ed.), *Speech evaluation in medicine.* Grune & Stratton.

Strominger, A., Winkler, M., & Cohen, L. (1984). Speech and language evaluation. In S. Pueschel (Ed.), *The young child with Down syndrome.* New York: Human Services Press.

Part II: Topics and Issues in Down Syndrome

14
Interdisciplinary Approaches

DON C. VAN DYKE AND FRANCES HEIDE

The clinical condition of Down syndrome was first described in 1866 in a paper published in the *London Hospital Reports* by the British neurologist, Dr. John Langdon Down. the clinical syndrome, however, has been with us for centuries, as indicated by 15th- and 17th-century paintings of children who appear to have phsyical characteristics of this syndrome (Patterson, 1987; Smith et al., 1976). The past literature dealing with theories of the etiology of this chromosomal syndrome is extensive (Pueschel & Steinberg, 1980). However, it was not until the cytogenetics work in the 1950s of Lejeune et al. that we had any real insight into the etiology of this syndrome. What was demonstrated was an extra number 21 chromosome in individuals with the clinical presentation of Down syndrome.

Current understanding of Down syndrome is that it is the phenotypic expression of a genotype that includes three copies of the q22 band of chromosome number 21. It has been estimated that chromosome 21 has 1,500 genes (Patterson, 1987). Most (95%) individuals with this syndrome are trisomic for the entire number 21 chromosome. Other persons with Down syndrome include those with translocations (3%) or significant mosaicism (2%) (Penrose & Smith, 1966). Down syndrome reflects the occurrence of a chromosomal anomaly that has the potential to afflict approximately one out of every 1,000 live births or 600 to 700 term pregnancies in the United States (Adam et al., 1981; Smith et al., 1976). The syndrome is prominently associated with mental retardation and is one of the major presenting diagnoses in both genetic and developmental clinics (de la Cruz & Gerald, 1981; Smith, 1982; Pueschel, 1983; Smith, 1982). Children with Down syndrome share some common features and yet are characterized by considerable variability in phenotypic expression and the effects of the genotypic excess on multiple organ systems (Scoggin & Patterson, 1982). For this reason, an *interdisciplinary* team approach has proven as useful with Down syndrome as with other developmental disorders. A *multidiscplinary* approach, in which knowledge from many fields is tapped, is common in the diagnosis and treatment of many disorders. A truly *interdisciplinary* approach, on the other hand, stresses not only the inclusion of professionals from a range of disciplines, but also the close cooperation of these professionals as they work to meet the needs and build the strengths of their patient.

Interdisciplinary concerns exist in other pediatric disorders, including cerebral palsy, myelomeningocele (spina bifida), cystic fibrosis, asthma, sickle cell anemia, nonspecific developmental delay, neurofibromatosis, and hemophilia. The incidence of cerebral palsy is 1:500 to 1:1000 births; of cystic fibrosis 1:2000; of spina bifida 1:1000 to 1:1200. It has been only recently that Down syndrome, with an equal or greater incidence, has been evaluated using an interdisciplinary approach that addresses the specific medical and educational needs of the child with Down syndrome.

The medical problems of Down syndrome are multiple, and these have a significantly impact on the provision of clinical care, family support systems, and the level of the child's participation in educational and developmental programs (Pueschel, 1983). The concept of an interdisciplinary approach to developmental delay, and the associated medical problems, is not new, but the application to Down syndrome of a combined preventive developmental/medical perspective is more recent. With the development of more diverse and appropriate medical experience and expertise and with the contributions derived from basic and clinical research, some of the preconceptions and possible misunderstandings related to Down syndrome are being remedied.

At least 27 interdisciplinary programs for Down syndrome are now operating in the continental United States and abroad (see Appendix 11). The development of an interdisciplinary approach to Down syndrome is based upon the realization that the special needs of children with Down syndrome require a coordinated interdisciplinary approach, not only in terms of developmental issues but also in regard to biomedical concerns. The clinical objectives of many interdisciplinary Down syndrome programs include:

1. Assistance and supplementation of the efforts of pediatricians, family physicians, psychologists, developmental centres, and educators in order to promote optimal development for children with Down syndrome.
2. Provision of superior preventive medical care to enhance the likelihood that each individual will realize her or his potential.

Some syndrome programs approach Down syndrome in a preventive medical model with subspecialty consultative services and a program devoted to clinical research. These programs are designed to meet the diverse needs of these individuals and their families and to provide a health-care program in one central location. Since children and adults with Down syndrome often manifest a variety of biomedical and developmental disorders, and since the birth of a Down syndrome child presents a family with a considerable challenge, it is essential to provide a source of consolidated specialized services, information, and counseling.

As expert medical care for individuals with Down syndrome is increasingly available, the mean life expectancy of these individuals will continue to increase, with more and more children surviving to adulthood. The concerns of pediatricians will become the problems of internists and family practice physicians. It should be a natural extension that programs for children with Down syndrome need to serve a transitional role, to extend needed services to adults with this disorder, and to provide support and education to the relevant health-care personnel, who in the future will provide primary medical care to these individuals.

Most interdisciplinary Down syndrome programs emphasize the initial provision of services to newborns and infants; however, children of all ages need such care. Often older individuals with Down syndrome were seen on an individual basis. The focus of adult Down syndrome programs is usually not only on biomedical disorders, but also upon rehabilitation and vocational needs.

The infant, toddler, and young adult portions of Down syndrome programs commonly focus on the needs of the parents, families, and individuals with Down syndrome. Included in the initial goals of these programs are the exploration of topics pertinent to Down syndrome and the development of information from which issues of special concern could be identified for further investigation.

Another goal of these programs is to provide information about Down syndrome to parents, professionals, and the general public. The use of computerized data retrieval by some programs has allowed for collection of relevant statistics, clinical correlation, and the study of multiple medical problems such as growth and nutrition, hearing and speech disorders, foot and gait problems, endocrinopathies, immune deficiency, infectious disease, ophthalmological problems, dental and craniofacial abnormalities, memory/cognitive deficits, and learning disabilities in Down syndrome.

The development of parent and professional groups by some of the programs has allowed for the creation of programs for public and professional education on the management of, and research relevant to, Down syndrome. As these programs progress, there is the potential for the provision of additional resources for the training of professionals from various disciplines in the medical, educational, nursing, psychology, dental, and other aspects of developmentally disabling disorders.

Summary

Interdisciplinary programs have been well received, providing as they do coordinated and efficient mechanisms for addressing multisystem disorders. It is felt that with the development of more diverse and appropriate medical expertise, and with the contributions derived from basic and clinical research, some of the preconceptions and misunderstandings relative to Down syndrome can be remediated. Interdisciplinary preventive health-care programs for individuals with this syndrome are likely to achieve the success that has marked other multifaceted programs, while also serving as resources for training professionals from various fields in aspects of developmentally disabling disorders of children and adults.

References

Adam, M.M., Erickson, J.D., Layde, P.M., & Oakley, G.P. (1981). Down's syndrome: Recent trends in the United States. *Journal of the American Medical Association, 246* (1), 758–760.

de la Cruz, F.F., & Gerald, P.S. (Eds.) (1981). *Trisomy 21 (Down syndrome) research perspective.* Baltimore: University Park Press.

Down, J.L.H. (1886). Observations on an ethnic classification of idiots, London Hospital. *Clinical Lecture and Reports, London Hospital, 3*, 259–262.

Lejeune, J., Gautier, M., & Turpin, R. (1959b). Études des chromosomes somatiques de neuf enfants mongoliens. *C.R. Acad of Science (Paris), 6* (248), 1721–1722.

Lejeune, J., Turpin, R., & Gautier, M. (1959). Le Mongolisme, prémier example d'aberration autosomique humaine. *Am. Genet. Paris, 1*, 41–49.

Patterson, D. (1987). The causes of Down syndrome. *Scientific American, 257* (2), 52–57.

Penrose, L.S., & Smith, G.F. (1966). *Down's anomaly.* London: J and A Churchill, Ltd.

Pueschel, S.M. (1983). The child with Down syndrome. In M.D. Levine, S.B. Carey, A.C. Crocker, & R.T. Gross (Eds.), *Developmental-behavioral pediatrics* (pp. 353–362). Philadelphia: W.B. Saunders.

Pueschel, S.M., & Steinberg, L. (1980). *Down syndrome: A comprehensive bibliography.* New York: Garland STPM Press.

Scoggin, C.H., & Patterson, D. (1982). Down's syndrome as a model disease. *Archives of Internal Medicine, 142* (3), 462–464.

Smith, G.F., & Berg, J.M. (1976). *Down's anomaly.* New York: Churchill-Livingstone Publishers.

Smith, D.W. (1982). *Decognizable Patterns of Human Malformations*, New York: W.B. Saunders.

15
Development and Behavior

Don C. Van Dyke, Marty Novak Hoffman,
Susan van Duyne, Frances Heide, and Ruth Zemke

Introduction

Much has been written about the developmental behavior of individuals with Down syndrome, particularly during the first three to five years of life. The literature demonstrates that a large number of these children demonstrate, in their first months, nearly normal development on such tests as the Bayley's Scale of Infant Development or the Vineland Adaptive Behavioral Scale. As time passes, relative performance levels decrease on these types of measures, sometimes provoking concern from parents, physicians, and educators. In general, it is known that children with Down syndrome demonstrate a wide varaition in mental and motor development. When comparing time of attainment of specific developmental milestones, such as the age at which a child is able to sit up, there is a much greater range for children with Down syndrome than for other children (Cunningham, 1982). The range of time of attainment for developmental milestones also increases with age among children with Down syndrome. Thus, it would seem that these children have slower rates of development and a greater amount of individual variation in rate which becomes more evident over time. It is as though different trajectories begin at nearly the same point, birth (with a limited behavioral repertoire), but "fan out" over time to produce an increasingly wider range, even if progress is ongoing.

Development in Down Syndrome

In a source book for parents (Cunningham, 1982), average ages of reaching various developmental milestones are listed for children with Down syndrome in comparison with other children (Appendices 2 and 3). This longitudinal study is primarily based on testing of over 150 children with Down syndrome. Cunningham reports the average age and range of ages at which a milestone is attained by children with Down syndrome, as compared to previously established developmental age ranges (Appendices 2 and 3). These developmental age ranges support the idea that children with Down syndrome have greater variability in developmental milestone attainment than other children, and this variability increases with age. An example of a milestone is sitting without support. A typical child attains this skill between the ages of 5 and 9 months (a 4-month range). Children with Down syndrome attain this milestone between 6 and 16 months (a 10-month range).

The increasing range of developmental attainment as the children grow older is shown in the more complex skill of walking alone. An average child attains this skill between 9 and 17 months (an 8-month range). A child with Down syndrome attains this skill between 13 and 48 months (a range of 35 months).

In fine motor and adaptive skills, this variability in developmental milestone attainment in children with Down syndrome is also shown. An average child can transfer objects between 4 and 8 months (a 4-month range); a child with Down syndrome transfers objects at between 6 and 12 months (a 6-month range).

Increasing age range of developmental attainments with age is shown in fine motor skills by the building of a tower of two cubes. An average child attains this skill between 10 and 19 months (a 9-month range). A child with Down syndrome attains this skill between 14 and 32 months (a range of 18 months).

Development of motor skills in children with Down syndrome has been studied by various authors (Carr, 1970; Schnell 1984). Generally, the research has indicated that motor skill development follows a normal, but slower, sequential progression than that of other children. Motor developmental attainments were studied with 89 infants by Zausmer and Shea (1984). The tool used for measuring development was an assessment scale formulated by Zausmer. This scale followed a normal developmental sequence and reflected both quantative and qualitative aspects of development. The quantitative aspect of test items referred to the attainment of a specific developmental skill (e.g., sitting unsupported); the qualitative aspect referred to how well the skill was performed (e.g., the degree of independence, the speed of peformance, the number of repetitions). The study concluded that motor development in children with Down syndrome followed a normal content and sequence of progression (e.g., sitting before walking). The difference was that children with this syndrome were slower in reaching the milestones. This slower rate was thought to be a result of hypotonia, hyperextensibility at the joints, congenital heart defects, and a decrease in muscle strength. All of these functions have a significant effect upon motor skills in humans. However, thhe specific impact of each of these functions on the motor development in children with Down syndrome has not been thoroughly explored. An example of how these functions affect motor development can be seen in the hyperextensibility and decreased muscle strength of the thumb. In combination, this can create a handicap in the ability to hold and manipulate small objects, a skill required in items measuring fine motor performance (Zausmer & Shea, 1984).

Schnell (1984) completed a longitudinal study of children with Down syndrome ($N = 78$–88) using the BSID, in which a decreasing level of performance with age was noted. Each child was assessed at semiannual visits, beginning at 6 months and continuing through 36 months of age. On the motor scale of the BSID, children with Down syndrome performed at between 53 and 67% of their chronological age norms. At 6 months, children with this syndrome performed at 67% of chronological age norms, while at 12 months they performed at 60% of chronological age norms. At 36 months, the performance level of these children had decreased to 53%.

Schnell (1984) believed this phenomenon could be attributed to the format used for many items on the BSID. Half of the items on the BSID used to determine appropriate development between the ages of 6 and 12 months involve sitting as a prerequisite. From 12 months through to the end of the test, 43 of the 49 remaining items involve some form of walking activity (standing on one foot, jumping off the ground). Schnell considered that this focus on sitting and walking skills (without using other motor skills in the test) contributes to the apparent deceleration of development when assessed using the psychomotor scale. However, these results were not specifically analyzed to determine significance.

The deceleration found by Schnell (1984) is supported by Carr (1970; see also chapter 10). In longitudinal measures of motor performance on the psychomotor scale of the BSID, Carr noted a general decline from birth to 10 months. While the decline continues, the rate of decline was less from 10 to 24 months.

The rate of motor development in children with Down syndrome and specific performance problems are affected by many factors. These factors are frequently seen in the form of secondary handicaps, such as hypotonia in children with neurological deficits. As with other disabilities, the issue is complicated because these factors affect all children to varying degrees. In children with Down syndrome, this is seen in muscle tone and subsequent extensibility of the joints. Sometimes the overall effect is further complicated by a heart defect. These factors are interrelated, making it difficult to observe one as distinct from the others (Schnell, 1984).

In general, research completed in the cognitive development of children with Down syndrome indicates that there will be some associated level of retardation (Cunningham, 1982). The intelligence of children with this syndrome generally falls within the range of moderate retardation (IQ 40–50). Early studies showed lower IQs, often in the range of severe retardation (IQ 20–30), but most of these earlier studies observed institutionalized children. IQ scores are known to be higher in children who are reared in the home and receive optimal treatment, developmental, and educational programs (Cunningham, 1982). Although retardation is expected, studies have been conducted of the mental and intellectual development of children with Down syndrome to determine whether their learning patterns are the same as that of other children.

Schnell (1984), in the study described previously, measured mental as well as motor functions. Schnell noted that the sample of children with DS ($N = 75$–88) scored slightly higher than half (55–58%) of the chronological age expectancy on the mental scale of the BSID when tested at 6-month age intervals for a period between 6 and 36 months. Mental scores showed less variability than the repeated measures of motor performance at different ages, and ranged from 53 to 67% of chronological age norms. In other words, Schnell did not find the deceleration in mental development that was found in motor development. In contrast, Carr (1970) found deceleration in both motor and mental development.

Carr (1970), in a longitudinal study previously cited, found a decline in the BSID mental scale scores similar to those reported for motor scale scores. In a more complete analysis, Carr (1975) also reported that the pattern of development in children with Down syndrome may possibly be different from the norm rather than just slower. Carr found that these children tended to stay at one stage longer (plateau for an extended period of time) than normal children. During longitudinal studies or in repeated measures for habilitation programs, these children's scores might appear to have fallen if they tested at the end of the plateau. This is possible because earlier in that stage the age discrepancy from normal may not have been as great as it was near the end of the plateau. Carr's 1975 test results were supported by informal comments made by mothers of children with Down syndrome. Mothers would frequently state that their children seemed to stay the same and that they did not think their children were going to do anything new. Then, all of a sudden, the children would perform some new skill. This observation, however, has not been validated by other studies concerned with the mental development of children with Down syndrome.

Morss (1983) explored the question of whether children with Down syndrome follow the same cognitive developmental sequence as other children, though progressing more slowly. A longitudinal study was conducted with two groups of infants, 8 with Down syndrome, and 26 without. An assessment scale was not used; instead, information was obtained on repeated longitudinal presentations of tasks. Six object-permanence tasks were used, comprising 3 pair of related items. These object-permanence tasks were used because information from previous studies had identified the successful and unsuccessful strategies used by children who did not have Down syndrome. Two sets of three trials were presented.

Morss (1983) found that cognitive development in children with Down syndrome is slow and progresses differently than that of other children. Infants with Down syndrome were less likely to repeat a success over time, demonstrating cause-and-effect learning relationships, than were other infants. Also, errors committed by the infants with Down syndrome were not characteristic of an error pattern predicted for each task, unlike other infants.

Silverstein, Legutki, Friedman, and Takayama (1982) completed a study with 377 institutionalized children with Down syndrome, with a comparison group made up of an equal number of children who did not have Down syndrome, but matched for chronological age, mental age, and age of institutionalization. All were tested with the Stanford-Binet Intelligence Scale, Form L or L-M. Results indicated that children with Down syndrome performed better on tasks that require figural content (shapes and concrete objects), and on visual-motor ability, when compared to other children. The items on which the other children performed better included semantic content (words and ideas), social intelligence, general comprehension, judgment, and reasoning. This study was limited to institutionalized children with Down syndrome, which affects the ability to generalize results. Studies have shown that institutionalized children with Down syndrome have lower mental age scores when compared to noninstitutionalized children with Down syndrome (Meindl et al., 1983). It is not known whether similar differences would be found between noninstitutionalized subjects matched for chronological age and developmental age.

Mental and intellectual growth in children with Down syndrome have been compared with normal growth and development. The results of some studies (Carr, 1970; Schnell, 1984) suggest that mental development is normal but slow. The linearity of the rate of mental development of children with Down syndrome is still not clear. While Schnell (1984) found a nearly linear relationship, Carr found a deceleration between 10 months and 2 years. More research is needed to determine the true picture. Some studies (Carr, 1975; Morss, 1983) indicate that mental development in children with Down syndrome is different from that of other children, and one study (Silverstein et al., 1982) found it to be different from other children with subnormal IQ levels who were matched for chronological and mental age with children with Down syndrome.

Comparisons of Mental and Motor Development

Studies have also been completed comparing the relationship of mental and motor development in children with Down syndrome. LaVeck and LaVeck (1977) used the BSID with 20 female and 20 male children with Down syndrome between the ages of 12 and 36 months. They established developmental quotients by applying the following equations: mental age equivalent/chronological age × 100. and psychomotor age equivalent chronological age × 100. They found that the mean mental quotients (66.06) were significantly higher than the mean motor quotients (53.11). The authors attributed this motor lag to hypotonia.

This study was then replicated with a younger population of children with Down syndrome (Harris, 1981). In the Harris study 20 children with Down syndrome (11 females, 9 males) between the ages of 2.7 months and 21.5 months were evaluated. The BSID were again administered. Results supported the findings of the LaVeck and LaVeck study in that mean mental quotients (82.79) were significantly higher than mean motor quotients (69.90) ($p < 0.05$), even with this younger sample. This study also demonstrated that the developmental disparity increases with age as previously stated. Harris found that the group of children in the study demonstrated a disparity between mental and motor skills of 1.54 months (mean chronological age of 10.2 months). LaVeck and LaVeck reported a lag between mental and motor skills of 2.86 months (mean chronological age of 22.2 months). A deceleration was noted with increasing chronological age as well as consistently superior mental performance over motor performance.

From the previous research cited in this study and from general knowledge of children with Down syndrome, the decreased developmental and subsequent functional levels of these children are apparent. Due to this disability, children with Down syndrome are continually encouraged to participate in programs designed to enhance their development.

Methods

Over a period of 18 months, a questionnaire was completed by 190 parents of infants, children, adolescents, and young adults with Down syndrome. The questionnaire asked specific questions regarding developmental milestones, behavior, and eating. On the questionnaire, a report of specific developmental milestones was asked of all parents. Those milestones were: smiling, rolling over, sitting alone, crawling, standing alone, and walking alone. Other milestones for which documentation was requested were using single words meaningfully, using short sentences, bladder training, bowel training, starting to feed her- or himself, and starting to dress her- or himself.

Specific questions were asked regarding speech therapy, physical therapy, occupational therapy, and research teaching. Inquiries were also made about counseling, tutoring, megavitamin therapy, and cell-therapy.

Behavior was determined using a behavioral checklist of eight items. The parents were asked whether their child was happy, playful, affectionate, and liked by other children. Other behavioral questions asked were whether the child was well-behaved with parents, well-behaved with brothers or sisters, as well-behaved in school in a normally active period.

The questionnaire was given to all 190 families; however, the response rate was not 100%. The number of responses received is denoted by *N*. The 190 individuals with Down syndrome were fairly evenly divided in regard to gender, with 48% male and 52% female. The age distribution showed that 25% were less than 1 year of age, 29% were between 1 and 3 years of age, 13% between 3 and 5 years of age, 22% between 5 and 12 years of age, and 11% between the ages of 12 and 21. In summary, two-thirds of the patient population was less than five years of age.

Developmental milestones by parental report are listed in Table 15.1, and show developmental milestones in approximately the same range as that

TABLE 15.1. Developmental milestones (by parental report).

	Male	Female
Smiling		
N[a]	72	85
Mean	11.8 wks 2.7 mo	8.8 wks 2 mo
STD dev	10.3 wks 2.4 mo	5.1 wks 1.2 mo
Rolling over		
N	66	81
Mean	16.4 wks 3.8 mo	17.9 wks 4.1 mo
STD dev	10.4 wks 2.4 mo	14.5 wks 3.3 mo
Sitting alone		
N	69	75
Mean	37.5 wks 8.7 mo	42.0 wks 9.7 mo
STD dev	16.6 wks 3.8 mo	28.6 wks 6.6 mo
Crawling		
N	63	60
Mean	53.4 wks 12.3 mo	61.5 wks 14.2 mo
STD dev	27.4 wks 3.8 mo	44.2 wks 10.3 mo
Standing alone		
N	53	52
Mean	95.1 wks 22 mo	82.9 wks 19.1 mo
STD dev	126.8 wks 29.3 mo	40.6 wks 9.4 mo
Walking alone		
N	58	53
Mean	127.3 wks 29.3 mo	105.7 wks 24.4 mo
STD dev	126.7 wks 29.2 mo	64.2 wks 14.8 mo
Using word meaning fully		
N	50	51
Mean	93.5 wks 21.6 mo	104.0 wks 24.0 mo
STD dev	69.6 wks 16.1 mo	86.5 wks 20.0 mo
Using short sentences		
N	30	30
Mean	210.7 wks 48.7 mo	184.9 wks 42.7 mo
STD dev	122.6 wks 28.3 mo	98.9 wks 22.8 mo
Bladder trained		
N	29	34
Mean	231.4 wks 53.4 mo	168.9 wks 30.0 mo
STD dev	143.8 wks 33.2 mo	95.1 wks 21.0 mo
Bowel trained		
N	28	31
Mean	193.7 wks 44.7 mo	182.3 wks 42.0 mo
STD dev	114.8 wks 26.5 mo	92.5 wks 21.4 mo
Starting to feed him/herself		
N	51	55
Mean	108.6 wks 25.1 mo	97.8 wks 22.6 mo
STD dev	75.6 wks 17.5 mo	97.4 wks 22.6 mo
Starting to dress him/herself		
N	32	35
Mean	240.4 wks 55.5 mo	225.7 wks 52.1 mo
STD dev	168.7 wks 39 mo	142.3 wks 32.9 mo

[a]N = number of completed responses.

TABLE 15.2. Resources provided (by parental report).

Resource	N[a]	Affirmative response[b]	Percent
Speech therapy (including signing)	183	118	64
Physical therapy	180	101	56
Occupational therapy	174	84	48
Resource teaching	163	28	17
Counseling	170	26	15
Tutoring	170	27	16
Megavitamin therapy	169	36	21
Cell therapy	177	21	12

[a]N = Number of completed responses to a questionnaire given to 190 parents of individuals with Down syndrome.
[b]To question, "What resources therapies were used?"

TABLE 15.3. Behavior (by parental report).

Identified behavior	N[a]	Affirmative parental responses	Percent
Happy child	186	181	97
Playful child	186	178	96
Affectionate child	179	170	95
Liked by other children	165	158	96
Well-behaved with parents	164	151	92
Well-behaved with sisters and brothers	132	119	90
Well-behaved in school	140	124	89

[a]N = Number of complete response to a questionnaire given to 190 parents of children with Down syndrome.

reported by Cunningham (1982) in Appendices 2 and 3. The table contains a number of items not used by Cunningham, and covers language and adaptive daily living (ADL) tasks, such as bowel/bladder training and feeding and dressing for both males and females. Thus, it records the overall parental perspective on both developmental and ADL skills for the older Down syndrome child.

In an effort to obtain a perspective of the parents' use of resources, parents were questioned as to whether they had ever had their child participate in traditional or nontraditional therapies. Almost two-thirds, or 64% of this patient population had received speech therapy and in some cases sign-language, 56% had received physical therapy, and 48% occupational therapy. Resource teaching, counseling, and tutoring were received by less than 20% of these individuals. In regard to nontraditional or alternative therapy, 21% were involved in some type of megavitamin therapy, and 12% (21 individuals) had received at least one or more injections of cell therapy.

Parental responses to the questions on behavior appear to support the generally held opinion that most children with Down syndrome are happy, affectionate and well-behaved. Ninety-five percent of these parents described their child as happy, playful, affectionate, and liked by other children. Over 90% described their children as well-behaved with their parents and brothers and sisters. Only 11% reported school problems.

Discussion

In general, it is felt that the children with Down syndrome follow the same developmental pattern as other children but tend to stay longer at a given stage. However, there is a wide range of variability. Children with this syndrome usually develop traditional ADL skills (such as bowel and bladder training, dressing and feeding, and expressive language), but at a significantly older age than other children. While many children with Down syndrome are involved in speech therapy, occupational therapy, and physical therapy, only a few are involved in special programs outside of the general school setting. A small but significant number of children are involved in alternative therapies. Behaviorally, these children are described by their parents as happy, affectionate, and mostly well-behaved, with only a small percentage reporting significant school problems.

Summary

Down syndrome children remain for a longer period of time at developmental stages, but show a wider variability at all stages than do non-Down syndrome children. There are, however, small differences between males and females (see Table 15.1). Most Down syndrome children are in developmental programs, with speech therapy the most common area of emphasis. Alternative therapies were seen in a small but significant number, with 21% receiving megavitamin therapy and 12% receiving cell therapy.

References

Carr, J. (1970). Mental and motor development in young Mongol children. *Journal of Mental Deficiency Research, 14* (3), 205–220.

Carr, J. (1975). *Young children with Down syndrome.* London: Buttersworths Publishers.

Cunningham, C. (1982). *Down's syndrome: An introduction for parents.* London: Souvenir Press.

Harris, S. (1981). Relationship of mental and motor development in Down's syndrome infants. *Physical and Occupational Therapy in Pediatrics, 1*, 13–18.

LaVeck, B., & LaVeck, G.D. (1977). Sex difference in development among young children with Down's syndrome. *Journal of Pediatrics, 91* (31), 767–769.

Meindl, J., Yater, A., Lamp, R., & Barclay, A. (1983). Mental growth of noninstitutionalized children with Down syndrome. *British Journal of Mental Subnormality, 29*, 50–56.

Morss, J.R. (1983). Cognitive development in the Down's syndrome infant: Slow or different? *British Journal of Educational Psychology, 53* (1), 40–47.

Schnell, R.R. (1984). Psychomotor development. In S. Pueschel (Ed.), *The young child with Down syndrome* (p. 207). New York: Human Sciences Press Inc.

Silverstein, A., Legutki, G., Friedman, S.L., & Takayama, D.L. (1982). Performance of Down syndrome individuals on the Stanford-Binet intelligence scale. *American Journal of Mental Deficiency, 86* (5), 548–554.

Zausman, E., & Shea, A. (1984). Motor development. In S. Pueschel (Ed.), *The young child with Down syndrome* (p. 143). New York: Human Sciences Press Inc.

16
Down Syndrome and Leukemia

ROBERT A. KRANCE AND DAVID J. LANG

Introduction

The coincidence of trisomy 21 and leukemia has interested clinicians since it was first reported by Brewster and Cannon (Brewster & Cannon, 1930). Although the understanding of both of these disorders has broadened since the first report of their association, new techniques in molecular biology and molecular genetics enhance the likelihood that the details of this relationship may soon be better understood. In this review, consideration will be given to the occurrence in Down syndrome of congenital leukemia, neonatal transient leukemoid reaction (alternative terms include neonatal myeloproliferative disorder, transient leukemia, pseudoleukemia), and acute leukemia. The epidemiology of leukemia in association with Down syndrome and the significance of this association to more general concerns in both Down syndrome and leukemia will be discussed. Finally, some areas for future research will be suggested.

Congenital Leukemia and Transient Leukemoid Reaction

In 1956, Krivit and Good provided epidemiologic data supporting the proposal that the simultaneous occurrence of Down syndrome and acute leukemia was more than coincidental. In a prior report of four children with Down syndrome and acute leukemia, the authors noted that "...these several cases of associated leukemia and mongolism must be taken to suggest that some biological relationship between the two diseases exists" (Krivit & Good, 1956).

By the use of questionnaires, Krivit and Good were able to document 66 co-incidental occurrences of Down syndrome and leukemia (Krivit & Good, 1956). Applying the most conservative estimates for the incidence of Down syndrome and the incidence of leukemia, the authors concluded that the coincidence of Down syndrome and leukemia was three times what was to be expected. More recent surveys, drawing from improved epidemiologic data, estimate the incidence of acute leukemia in Down syndrome children to be 10–20 times that of non-Down syndrome children (Miller, 1969; Evans & Steward, 1972; Robinson et al., 1984).

Serendipitous information obtained from the questionnaire of Krivit and Good suggested a high frequency of congenital leukemia among infants with Down syndrome. Miller confirmed the incidence of congenital leukemia to be increased among neonates with Down syndrome. Based upon information extracted from death certificates, Miller estimated that one in every five or six newborns with congenital leukemia would also be a Down syndrome infant. Miller noted that this exceeded the frequency of Down syndrome in older children with leukemia, which he estimated as 1:36 (Miller, 1969). Corroborative data regarding the heightened frequency of neonatal leukemia and Down syndrome remain limited. A more recent epidemiologic survey investigating cause of death among the age group 20 to 34 years, established that the increased risk for leukemia in Down syndrome extends into adulthood (Schnoll, Stein, & Hansen, 1982). In this survey, however, no excess leukemic deaths were noted among children with Down syndrome under one year of age. The data base consisted of death certificates for a single year. The data were censored by removal of those death certificates in which Down syndrome was recorded as the underlying rather than the contributory cause of death (nearly 20% of the certificates). The impact of this manipulation cannot be assessed. Other reports, however, do acknowledge that the frequency of congenital leukemia in association with Down syndrome exceeds the expected rate (Fong & Brodeur, 1987; Rosner & Lee, 1972).

Compounding the difficulty in determining the true frequency of Down syndrome and congenital leukemia is the phenomenon of transient leukemoid reaction. First recognized by Ross (1963), this syndrome exhibits many features of congenital leukemia and may easily be misdiagnosed as such. The infant boy with Down syndrome described by Ross presented at 8 days of age with enlargement of the liver and spleen, elevated white count, and 28% myeloblasts in the white blood cell differential (Ross, Moloney, & Desforges, 1963). Hemoglobin and platelet count were initially satisfactory. Examination of the bone marrow demonstrated all three hematopoietic cell lines, but platelet and red cell precursors were reduced and the percentage of myeloblasts was excessive. The infant received a two-week course of drug therapy, after which the white cell count gradually declined to normal. By four months of age, the blood and bone marrow parameters were normal. When the child died at 3-3/4 years of age from unrelated causes, autopsy findings excluded leukemia. Although the original diagnosis was acute or subacute granulocytic leukemia, Ross reasoned that the diagnosis was incorrect because it was "...extremely unlikely that a remission of such long duration could occur without specific therapy and with completely normal findings both at follow-up and at autopsy" (Ross et al., 1963). It was speculated that perhaps in Down syndrome there is ineffective regulation of the production or maturation of leukocytes in response to an unknown stimulant: "...the child with

Mongolism may respond excessively with a non-fatal disorder resembling acute granulocytic leukemia..." (Ross et al., 1963). "Moreover, such an abnormality would conceivably make Mongoloid children more susceptible to the factor or factors which result in true leukemia" (Ross et al., 1963).

The work of Rosner and Lee helped to clarify the information relative to Down syndrome, neonatal leukemia, and transient leukemoid reaction (1972). They identified nine infants with Down syndrome in a group of infants diagnosed with acute leukemia. However, after evaluating case records, only two of these nine infants could be confirmed as having leukemia. In three patients the "leukemia" resolved spontaneously in a matter of weeks, a clinical behavior not compatible with leukemia. For the other four infants, the diagnosis of leukemia could neither be verified nor refuted. The authors also reviewed the medical literature, finding 47 instances of newborns with Down syndrome and leukemia. In eighteen of these newborns, the course following diagnosis was more compatible with transient leukemoid reaction. For the 29 infants with congenital leukemia, Rosner and Lee noted that acute myeloblastic leukemia was the more common variant, present in almost 60% of the cases, with acute lymphoblastic leukemia comprising the remaining cases. The preponderance in Down syndrome congenital leukemia of the acute myeloblastic morphotype parallels the distribution in non-Down syndrome congenital leukemia (Weinstein, 1978). Rosner and Lee cautioned that among the 18 newborns with Down syndrome having the transient leukemoid reaction, 14 were myeloblastic in appearance.

For infants with Down syndrome, the distinction between transient leukemoid reaction and congenital leukemia is crucial. In the case of transient leukemoid reaction, the passage of time and the judicious use of supportive measures often result in restoration of the normal hematopoietic state. On the other hand, without effective anti-leukemic chemotherapy, congenital leukemia is invariably fatal, and delay in initiating treatment may obviate its potential benefit. Recent improvements in the treatment of congenital leukemia have given rise to optimism (Reaman et al., 1987). This has made the necessity of distinguishing between congenital leukemia and transient leukemoid reaction even more acute.

Rosner and Lee (1972) noted that in 18 of 22 cases of Down syndrome and transient leukemoid reaction signs or symptoms were manifest in the newborn period, that is, at less than one month of age. Findings that suggest leukemia but are not apparent in the first month increase the likelihood that this is true leukemia. Infants with congenital leukemia present with skin nodules in up to 50% of cases (Weinstein, 1978). This feature is rarely reported in transient leukemoid reaction. Transient leukemoid reaction has occurred in the setting of ABO or Rh immunohemolytic diesase, pulmonary infections, cyanotic heart disease, cirrhosis, and congenital infection (Rosner & Lee, 1972; Weinstein, 1978). The relationship between transient leukemoid reaction and these other disorders is uncertain, but these associations emphasize the caution proffered by Ross (vide supra). In the end, however, distinction between congenital leukemia and transient leukemoid reaction on a clinical basis remains problematic. Most pediatric hematologists prefer watchful waiting in such circumstances, supporting the infant with appropriate measures and delaying chemotherapy until the true leukemic course becomes evident. In this regard, most troubling are the reports of Down syndrome newborns with transient leukemoid reaction who then later in life develop acute leukemia (Honda, Punnett, Charney, Miller & Thiede, 1964; Lin, Menaka, Lin, & Yong, 1980). Such occurrences ultimately blur the distinction between the two entities.

What relationship exists between congenital leukemia and transient leukemoid reaction? What are the factors that promote the leukemoid response? Why is this disordered myelopoiesis seen almost exclusively in infants with Down syndrome? Answers to these questions will complement the current understanding of the mechanisms that control myelopiesis and hematopoiesis. Weinberger and Olenick (1970) established that newborns with Down syndrome may manifest disordered hematopoiesis involving not only white cells but red cells and platelets as well. From blood samples collected on over 44,000 newborns, 402 infants were identified as polycythemic (defined as hematocrit value exceeding the mean hematocrit by two standard deviations). Nine of these 402 polycythemic infants were phenotypically classified as Down syndrome. Based upon age-matched controls, the authors concluded that infants with Down syndrome were 19.2 times more likely to be polycythemic. Miller and Cosgriff (1983) found that among 61 cytogenetically confirmed Down syndrome newborns, 28 (45%) demonstrated some abnormality in the blood count. Most common was an increase in hematocrit, but four infants with Down syndrome had a decrease in platelet count; one of these had a concurrent elevation in white count. Three infants manifested both a decrease in platelet count and an increase in hematocrit. Beyond the immediate newborn period, myelofibrosis, myeloid metaplasia, and aplastic anemia have been described in children with Down syndrome (Rosner & Lee, 1972; Weinblatt, Higgins, & Ortega, 1981). The hematologic spectrum that occurs in Down syndrome newborns is broad. It remains to be determined whether this spectrum actually is a continuum, with a normal blood count and neonatal leukemia comprising the extremes, or whether these variations are separate and distinct.

In vitro cell culture of leukemic cells has been widely used to study leukemia cell biology. When compared to normal hematopoietic cells, leukemic cells fail to develop the colonies and clusters that are typical of normal hematopoietic growth (Moore, Spitzer, Williams, Metcalf, & Buckley, 1974). As a potential application of this observation, cell culture techniques have been employed to differentiate between acute leukemia and transient leukemoid reaction in Down syndrome. Unfortunately, the results of these efforts have not proven definitive. Denegri reported on the in vitro growth characteristics of blood and bone marrow obtained from three Down syndrome newborns with transient leukemoid reaction (Denegri, Rogers, Chan, Sadoway, & Thomas,

1981). Normal in vitro growth was obtained in each case. A striking finding of this study was that maternal post-partum serum added to the culture system caused marked growth inhibition of infant's bone marrow. Maternal serum also inhibited in vitro growth of bone marrow from unrelated healthy donors and cryopreserved leukemic cells. This inhibitory activity was not thought to be immunologically mediated. The factor responsible for inhibition was no longer present in maternal sera obtained two months post-partum. Only weak inhibition of in vitro growth was found using control post-partum serum in identical experiments. Barak et al. (1982), also found normal in vitro growth of bone marrow cells from an infant with Down syndrome and transient leukemoid reaction; but under similar circumstances, other investigators report both atypical and abnormal in vitro growth (Mendelow, Krawitz, Cohn, & Bernstein, 1984; Wong, Jones, Srivastava, & Gruppo, 1985; Coulombel et al., 1987). In one study, the in vitro growth in a Down syndrome newborn with transient leukemoid reaction was indistinguishable from the type of growth associated with acute leukemia (Mendelow, 1984). In spite of this, the abnormal hematologic findings resolved. The authors cautioned that the decision to treat such a patient with chemotherapy should not be predicated upon in vitro growth patterns (Coulombel, 1987). A more recent study of two neonates with Down syndrome and transient leukemoid reaction demonstrated that both normal and abnormal, "leukemic," in vitro growth occurred coincidentally. Moreover, as the patients' blood picture normalized, the cell culture assays correspondingly became free of abnormal colonies and clusters. This report and one other noted that the abnormal in vitro growth returned when these patients developed acute leukemia (Wong et al., 1987). Given that a portion of infants with Down syndrome and transient leukemoid reaction subsequently develop leukemia, perhaps this regression/progression of abnormal in vitro growth is to be expected.

Improved cytogenetic techniques have helped to clarify the relationships between Down syndrome, transient leukemoid reaction, and leukemia. Evidence now suggests that genetic information present on chromosome 21 may be a crucial determinant of disordered hematopoiesis. In an illustrative case, a phenotypically normal newborn child was noted to have a markedly elevated white blood cell count, 136,000/mm3 with 70% myeloblasts (Brodeur, Dahl, Williams, Tipton, & Kalwinsky, 1980). Karyotype determination performed on blood and bone marrow was almost exclusive for +21. Conversely, just 4% skin fibroblast karyotypes were +21; the remainder were normal. The infant's hematologic picture normalized without therapy. Repeat cytogenetic studies on bone marrow and blood 100 days post-partum, demonstrated almost complete reversal of the earlier karyotype findings. The implication is that the extra chromosome was responsible for transient leukemoid reaction. A similar report has been made by Heaton, Fitzgerald, Fraser, & Abbot (1981).

Rowley (1981) proposed that the extra chromosome 21 is a critical factor predisposing to development of acute leukemia in patients with Down syndrome. Three observations were offered to support this hypothesis. First, in patients with acute lymphoblastic leukemia (ALL) and acute nonlymphoblastic leukemia (ANLL), +21 is the most common cytogenetic abnormality. The highest frequency of +21 is among children with ALL; 31% of children with ALL who have an abnormal karyotype will have +21. Since +21 is more common in ALL than in ANIL and since ALL occurs more commonly in children, +21 in some way predisposes to ALL. Finally, when transient leukemoid reaction occurs in phenotypically normal but genotypically mosaic +21 children, the proliferating clone is uniformly +21. Upon resolution of transient leukemoid reaction, there is concurrent diminishment of the trisomic clone. This hypothesis that +21 is teleologically involved in leukemia has been criticized principally for relating chromosomal changes in leukemic (cancerous) cells of non-Down syndrome patients to a constitutional abnormality that occurs in all cells of children with trisomy 21. Not all children with Down syndrome develop leukemia, and only a portion of non-Down syndrome patients with acute leukemia manifest +21 leukemic genotype (Fong & Brodeur, 1987). In transient leukemoid reaction the myeloproliferative picture is almost always myeloblastic, while the most common leukemia among Down syndrome children is acute lymphoblastic leukemia. The mere presence of +21 cannot totally account for the onset of malignancy. Nonetheless, the association between +21 and leukemoid and leukemic events appears more than coincidental.

The assumption that the extra 21 chromosome or a critical fragment thereof may be casually related to the development of leukemia seems correct. Perhaps the extragenetic material in patients with Down syndrome increases susceptibility to mutagenic factors. It has been demonstrated that Down syndrome cells grown in culture and infected by oncogenic virus are transformed more readily than fibroblasts from non-Down syndrome individuals (Todaro & Martin, 1967). This tendency to morphologic and malignant transformation (aberrant in vitro growth pattern) has been seen in cell lines derived from patients with other genetically determined conditions that in addition demonstrate an increased susceptibility to malignancy. It has been shown that trisomy 21 cells are more susceptible to X-ray induced genetic damage and that repair of sublethal X-ray damage in these trisomic cells differs from repair in normal cells (Countryman, Heddle, & Crawford, 1977). Thus, there is evidence that certain known mutagens demonstrate greater activity in trisomy 21 cells. These observations have not undergone recent scrutiny. With the recognition of oncogenes and the search for the relative mechanism associated with malignant transformation, the interplay of extragenetic material and oncogenes needs to be explored. Alternatively, gene(s) on chromosome 21 may act to unmask or repress known or even as-yet-undefined oncogenes located in other chromosomes. Ultimately, the underlying basis for malignancy must lie in the area of genetic control. In this case, therefore, it would not be surprising that a genetic imbalance, such as trisomy or translocation, might influence the occurrence of some form of cancer.

It is to be expected that an enhanced understanding of how genetic errors occur and are expressed will permit modification or prevention of disorders, whether at the cellular level, as in leukemia, or as expressed in the totality of the individual as in Down syndrome.

Acute Leukemia

Acute leukemia has been documented to occur in both nondisjunction and translocation Down syndrome; whether the leukemic predilection is similar for both is unknown (Fong & Brodeur, 1987; Hecht, Hecht, Morgan, Sandberg, & Link, 1986). The preponderance of ALL over ANLL among children, 70–80% vs 20–30%, is maintained in Down syndrome patients with acute leukemia (Robinson et al., 1984; Rosner & Lee, 1972). The peak age of incidence in childhood ALL and Down syndrome children with ALL is also similar, 5.8 years and 6.2 years, respectively. In contrast, among Down syndrome patients with ANLL the age at diagnosis was significantly younger than it was among non-Down syndrome patients. Seventy-five percent were younger than three years in the Robinson series; in Rosner's report the median age at diagnosis for Down syndrome patients was two years. Unlike in older children, congenital leukemia is predominantly ANLL. Down syndrome children follow this distributive pattern. Because of the high frequency of congenital leukemia in Down syndrome, the earlier age of onset for ANLL among Down syndrome children may be explained by this phenomenon.

In treating children with Down syndrome and ALL, recent results permit optimism (Robinson et al., 1984). Although overall survival was somewhat less in Down syndrome children as compared to non-Down syndrome patients, event-free survival was the same-approximately 50%. This implies that Down syndrome ALL patients may expect treatment results comparable to non-Down syndrome patients. The higher mortality rate among Down syndrome patients during remission induction therapy, which accounts for the reduced overall survival, is offset by a lower relapse rate during later phases of treatment. When analyzed for the presence of clinical or laboratory features that predict poor response to treatment (e.g., high initial white count, older age, unfavorable leukemic cell surface markers), the frequency of these features in Down syndrome patients was similar to that of non-Down syndrome patients. However, Down syndrome children with ALL do experience more toxicity related to chemotherapy. In general, this added toxicity is due to exaggeration of the usual side effects of chemotherapy rather than to idiosyncracies peculiar to Down syndrome children. For example, Down patients were more likely to develop hyperglycemia while receiving L-asparaginase (Kalwinsky, Pui, & Bowman, 1982). More problematic for Down syndrome ALL patients was chemotherapy-induced myelosuppression. In one report, chemotherapy-induced leukopenia was more severe in Down children and often necessitated dose reduction (Blatt,

Albo, Prinn, Orlando, & Wollman, 1986). A possible explanation for this observation was the finding that, compared to an appropriate control, a group of Down syndrome children with ALL sustained significantly higher plasma drug concentration 42 hours post treatment with methotrexate (Garre et al., 1987). Development of severe gastrointestinal and hematologic toxicity correlated with these higher plasma methotrexate concentrations. A fuller understanding of the altered chemotherapy pharmacokinetics in Down syndrome patients may improve the results of their treatment.

Although avoiding undue drug toxicity is desirable, even more important is the administration of effective doses of chemotherapy to children who have relapsed with ALL. Leukemic relapse was once a fatal pronouncement; newer more aggressive therapies, including bone marrow transplantation, now salvage such patients (Rivera, Kovnar, et al., 1987; Rivera, George, et al., 1986; Rivera, Buchanan, et al., 1986; Sanders et al., 1985). The initial report of Down syndrome patients undergoing bone marrow transplantation was pessimistic (Rubin, O'Leary, Koch, & Nesbit, 1986). Only one of four patients survived, and every patient developed severe toxicity related to the bone marrow transplant preparatory regimen. Subsequently, with the development of transplant preparatory regimens which avoid total body irradiation, Down syndrome patients have successfully undergone this procedure (Tutschka, Copelan, & Klein, 1987; Wong et al., 1987).

Among Down syndrome children with ANLL, the uncommon morphotypes, acute megakaryoblastic and acute erythroblastic leukemia, have been reported in addition to the more common myeloblastic and monoblastic types (Villeval et al., 1986; Zipursky, Peeters, & Poon, 1987). Whether these rare variants are represented disproportionately among Down patients is uncertain. If this proves to be true, therapy will need to be specifically adapted to morphotype. Among a presumably heteregenous group of ANLL patients with Down syndrome, Robinson found the treatment outcome comparable to that of other patients. Unfortunately, the results of treatment were unsatisfactory with overall survival less than 25%. Newer and generally more aggressive treatment regimens, including BMT, have improved disease-free survival in children with ANLL (Weinstein, Mayer, Rosenthal, et al., 1983; Brochstein, Kernan, Groshen, et al., 1987).

Summary

The frequency of acute leukemia in individuals with Down syndrome is 10–20 times higher than the incidence in the general population. In addition to the higher occurrence of leukemia (including congenital leukemia) infants with Down syndrome may also manifest transient leukemoid reaction. Transient leukemoid reaction may be misdiagnosed as leukemia but will in virtually every case resolve spontaneously. The dilemma is that untreated congenital leukemia is invariably fatal. This indicates the importance of distinguishing these conditions. Additional related and unrelated disorders of hematopoiesis also occur with an increased frequency in persons with Down syndrome.

This chapter reviews these issues and makes reference to the current experience with management of and outlook for children with Down syndrome who experience these conditions. The occurrence of leukemia is of course not limited to those with Down syndrome but, in addition to its more frequent occurrence, leukemia in persons with Down syndrome poses some therapeutic problems. The fact that the extra number 21 chromosome predisposes to an increase in the frequency of leukemia presents challenges in management, but also provides unique opportunities for the study of Down syndrome as well as of leukemia. Reference is made to investigative efforts and concepts, as well as to the current experience with therapy. This chapter has undergone several revisions in the past 2 years and even during this relatively brief time there has been a significant and favorable evolution in the success attendant upon treatment of persons with Down syndrome and leukemia. Further progress in understanding and therapy can certainly be anticipated.

References

Barak, Y., Mogilner, B.M., Karov, Y., Nir, E., Schlesinger, M., & Levin, S. (1982). Transient acute leukemia in a newborn with Down's syndrome. *Acta Paediatr Scand, 71*, 699–701.

Blatt, J., Albo, V., Prinn., V., Orlando, S., & Wollman, M. (1986). Excessive chemotherapy-related myelotoxicity in children with Down syndrome and acute lymphoblastic leukemia. *Lancet, 2*, 914.

Brewster, H.F., & Cannon, H.E. (1930). Acute lymphatic leukemia: report of a case in eleventh month Mongolian idiot. *New Orleans Medical and Surgical Journal, 82*, 872–873.

Brochstein, J.A., Kernan, N.A., Groshen, S., Cirrincione, C., Shank, B., Emanuel, D., Laver, J., & O'Reilly, R.J. (1987). Allogeneic bone marrow transplantation after hyperfractionated total-body irradiation and cyclophosphamide in children with acute leukemia. *The New England Journal of Medicine, 317*, 1618–1624.

Brodeur, G.M., Dahl, G.V., Williams, D.L., Tipton, R.E., & Kalwinsky, D.K. (1980). Transient leukemoid reaction and trisomy 21 mosaicism in phenotypically normal newborn. *Blood, 55*, 691–693.

Coulombel, L., Dercycke, M., Villeval, J.L., Leonard, C., Breton-Gorius, J., Vial, M., Bourgeois, P., & Tchernia, G. (1987). Characterization of the blast cell population in two neonates with Down's syndrome and transient myeloproliferative disorder. *British Journal of Haematology, 66*, 69–76.

Countryman, P.I., Heddle, J.A., & Crawford, E. (1977). The repair of X-ray induced chromosomal damage in trisomy 21 and normal diploid lymphocytes. *Cancer Research, 37*, 52–58.

de Alarcon, P.A., Patel, S., Goldberg, J., Allen, J.B., & Shaw, S. (1987). Infants with Down's syndrome. *Cancer, 60*, 987–993.

Denegri, J.F., Rogers, P.C.J., Chan, K.W., Sadoway, J., & Thomas, J.W. (1981). In vitro cell growth in neonates with Down's syndrome and transient myeloproliferative disorder. *Blood, 58*, 675–677.

Evans, D.K., & Steward, J.K. (1972). Down's syndrome and leukemia. *Lancet*, 2, 1322.

Fabil, J., & Drolette, M. (1970). Malformations and leukemia in children with Down's syndrome. *Pediatrics, 45*, 60–70.

Fong, C., & Brodeur, G.M. (1987). Down syndrome and leukemia: Epidemiology, genetics, cytogenetics and mechanisms of leukemogenesis. *Cancer Genet Cytogenet, 28*, 55–76.

Garre, M.L., Relling, M.V., Kalwinsky, D., Dodge, R., Crom. W.R., Abromowitch, M., Pui, C.H., & Evans, W.E. (1987). Pharmacokinetics and toxicity of methotrexate in children with Down syndrome and acute lymphocytic leukemia. *Journal of Pediatrics, 111*, 606–612.

Heaton, D.C., Fitzgerald, P.H., Fraser, G.J., & Abbott, G.D. (1981). Transient leukemoid proliferation of the cytogenetically unbalanced +21 cell line of a constitutionally mosaic boy. *Blood, 57*, 883–887.

Hecht, R., Hecht, B.K., Morgan, R., Sandberg, A.A., & Link, M.P. (1986). Chromosome clues to acute leukemia in Down syndrome. *Cancer Genet Cytogenet, 21*, 93–98.

Honda, F., Punnett, H.H., Charney, E., Miller, G., & Thiede, H.A. (1964). Serial cytogenetic and hematologic studies on a Mongol with trisomy–21 and acute congenital leukemia. *Journal of Pediatrics, 65*, 880–887.

Kalwinsky, D., Pui, C.H., & Bowman, W.P. (1982). Acute lymphocytic leukemia in children with Down syndrome. *Proceedings of the American Society of Clin Onco, 1*, 126.

Krivit, W., & Good, R.A. (1956). The simultaneous occurrence of leukemia and Mongolism: Report of four cases. *American Journal of Diseases of Children, 91*, 218–222.

Lin, H.P., Menaka, H., Lim, K.H., & Yong, H.S. (1980). Congenital leukemoid reaction followed by fatal leukemia. *American Journal of Diseases of Children, 134*, 939–941.

Mendelow, B., Krawitz, S., Cohn, R., & Bernstein, R. (1984). "Leukemic" pattern of in vitro growth in a patient with Down syndrome and transient myeloproliferative disorder. *American Journal of Hematology, 16*, 293–296.

Miller, M., & Cosgriff, M.J. (1983). Hematologic abnormalities in newborn infants with Down syndrome. *American Journal of Medical Genetics, 16*, 172–177.

Miller, R.W. (1969). Childhood cancer and congenital defects: A study of U.S. death certificates during the period 1960–1966. *Pediatrics Research, 3*, 389–397.

Miller, R.W. (1970). Neoplasia and Down's syndrome. *Annals of the New York Academy of Science, 171*, 637–644.

Miller, R.W., & Fraumeni, J.F. (1968). Down's syndrome and neonatal leukemia. *Lancet, 2*, 404.

Moore, M.A.S., Spitzer, G., Williams, N., Metcalf, D., & Buckley, J. (1974). Agar culture studies in 127 cases of untreated acute leukemia: The prognostic value of reclassification of leukemia according to in vitro growth characteristics. *Blood, 44*, 1–18.

Reaman, G.H., Steinberg, P.G., Gaynon, P.S., Bleyer, W.A., Finkelstein, J.Z., Evans, R., Miller, D.R., Sather, H.N., & Hammond, G.D. (1987). Improved survival of infants less than one-year of age with acute lymphoblastic leukemia treated with intensive multiagent chemotherapy. *Cancer Treatment Reports, 71*, 1033–1038.

Rivera, G.K., Buchanan, G., Boyett, J.M., Camitta, B., Ochs, J., Kalwinsky, D., Amylon, M., Vietti, T.J., & Crist, W.M. (1986). Intensive treatment of childhood acute lymphoblastic leukemia in first bone marrow relapse, Pediatric Oncology Group study. *New England Journal of Medicine, 315*, 273–278.

Rivera, G.K., George, S.H., Williams, D., Look, A.T., Abromowitch, M., Pui, C.H., Ochs, J.J., Dahl, G.V., Kalwinsky, D.K., Mirro, J., Dow, L.W., Raimondi, S., & Murphy, S.B. (1986). Early results of intensified remission induction chemotherapy for childhood acute lymphyocytic leukemia. *Medical Pediatric Oncology, 14*, 177–181.

Rivera, G.K., Kovnar, E., Pui, C.H., Dahl, G.V., Abromowitch, M., Ochs, J.J., Look, A.T., Kalwinsky, D.K., Mirro, J., Dow, L.W., & Murphy, S.B. (1987). Limiting toxicities during intensified remission induction chemotherapy for childhood acute lymphocytic leukemia. *Hamatol Bluttransfus, 30*, 156–160.

Robinson, L.L., Nesbit, M.E., Sather, H.N., Level, C., Shahidi, N., Kennedy, A., & Hammond, D. (1984). Down syndrome and acute leukemia in children: A 10 year retrospective survey from Children's Cancer Study Group. *Journal of Pediatrics, 105*, 235–242.

Rosner, F., & Lee, S.L. (1972). Down's syndrome and acute leukemia: Myeloblastic or lymphoblastic? Report of 43 cases and review of the literature. *American Journal of Medicine, 53*, 203–218.

Ross, J.D., Moloney, W.C., & Desforges, J.F. (1963). Ineffective regulation of granulopoieses masquerading as congenital leukemia in a mongoloid child. *Journal of Pediatrics, 63*, 1–10.

Rowley, J.D. (1981). Down syndrome and acute leukaemia: Increased risk may be due to trisomy 21. *Lancet, 2*, 1020–1022.

Rubin, C.M., O'Leary, M., Koch, P.A., & Nesbit, M.E., Jr. (1986). Bone marrow transplantation for children with acute leukemia and Down syndrome. *Pediatrics, 78*, 688–691.

Sanders, J.E., Flournoy, N., Thomas, E.D., Buckner, C.D., Lum, L.G., Clift, R.A., Appelbaum, F.R., Sullivan, K.M., Stewart, P., Deeg, H.J., Doney, K., & Storb, R. (1985). Marrow transplant experience in children with acute lymphoblastic leukemia: An analysis of factors associated with survival, relapse, and graft-versus-host disease. *Medical Pediatric Oncology, 13*, 165–172.

Schnoll, T., Stein, Z., & Hansen, H. (1982). Leukemia and other cancers, anomalies and infections as causes of death in Down syndrome in the United States during 1976. *Developmental Medical Child Neurology, 24*, 817–829.

Todaro, G.J., & Martin, G.M. (1967). Increased susceptibility of Down's syndrome fibroblasts to transformation by SV40. *Proceedings of the Society of Experimental Biology and Medicine, 124*, 1232–1236.

Tutschka, P.J., & Copelan, E.A., & Klein, J.P. (1987). Bone marrow transplantation for leukemia following a new busulfan and cyclophosphamide regimen. *Blood, 70*, 1382–1388.

Villeval, J.L., Cramer, P., Lemoine, F., Henri, A., Bettaieb, A., Bernaudin, F., Beuzard, Y., Berger, R., Flandrin, G., Breton-Gorius, J., & Vainchenker, W. (1986). Phenotype of early erythroblastic leukemias. *Blood, 68*, 1167–1174.

Weinberger, M.W., & Olenick, A. (1970). Congenital marrow dysfunction in Down's syndrome. *Journal of Pediatrics, 77*, 273–279.

Weinblatt, M.E., Higgins, G., & Ortega, J.A. (1981). Aplastic anemia in Down's syndrome. *Pediatrics, 67*, 896–897.

Weinstein, H. (1978). Congenital leukaemia and the neonatal myeloproliferative disorders associated with Down's syndrome. *Clin in Haematology, 7*, 147–154.

Weinstein, H.J., Mayer, R.J., Rosenthal, D.S., Coral, F.S., Camitta, B.M., & Gelber, R.D. (1983). Chemotherapy for acute myelogenous leukemia in children and adults: VAPA update. *Blood*, 62, 315–319.

Wong, K.Y., Jones, M.M., Srivastava, A.K., & Gruppo, R.A. (1987). Transient myeloproliferative disorder and acute nonlymphoblastic leukemia in Down syndrome. *Journal of Pediatrics*, 112, 18–22.

Zipursky, A., Peeters, M., & Poon, A. (1987). Megakaryoblastic leukemia and Down syndrome: A review. *Prog Clinical Biol Research*, 246, 33–56.

17
Issues of Family Interaction, Parenting, and Parent Groups

SUSAN VAN DUYNE, TONI MONSON, AND FRANCES HEIDE

Introduction

At the birth of a Down syndrome child, a family must consider a number of unexpected issues: parental reactions to the diagnosis of Down syndrome and its associated developmental disabilities, interfamilial relationships such as those between siblings, relationships with the extended family, and the role of professionals in facilitating family adjustment (Cobb & Hancock, 1984). The marital relationship, individual personalities, coping strategies, and financial situation will all affect the family's adjustment to the birth of a child with Down syndrome (Burden, 1980). Many studies in the literature have sought to determine the psychological variables that will predict the pattern of family adjustment to the birth of a child with a developmental disability. However, a review of this literature reveals that no currently available behavioral or psychological instrument measures or evaluates family stress following the birth of a disabled child or the relationship of these early levels of stress to later levels of adjustment by the family (A Murphy, 1982).

In a study involving 190 individuals with Down syndrome, one or both parents were interviewed by a psychologist and, in most cases, by a social worker. Efforts to develop an instrument to identify specific variables of family stress were not successful. At the present time, no variable(s) or questionnaire(s) seem to be of much assistance in assessing the level of stress in the family (A Murphy, 1982). However, the efforts to compile variables has resulted in the development of a checklist of issues (Table 16.1).

The First Year

Ambivalence, sadness, and disappointment by parents toward a child with Down syndrome are common (Vaisbren, 1980). Dealing with these emotions is a dynamic process; parental attitudes, hopes, expectations, and concern about their child change daily as they cope with their own emotions and progress at their own pace through various stages of their development (A.

Murphy, 1982). Some parents deal with feelings in a short period of time while others never come to grips with their emotions and never reach an acceptance of the situation. For some parents, passage of the first birthday of the child may spell the turning point. As one parent writes, "Until Laurie was one year old she was, in our mind, a Down syndrome child. Down syndrome was her major feature. After her first birthday she became a child...who had Down syndrome."

The mother of a newborn with Down syndrome writes, "Nobody ever said anything about feelings. The grief has lasted and lasted and it has its greedy grasp upon my soul. How can I handle it in the future when people stare at my child? There is an ebb and flow to our sadness. My immediate response was disbelief and adamant denial." She articulates many of the feelings and emotions that parents of children with Down syndrome initially feel. These parents must deal with the acceptance of the diagnosis, fatigue, depression, guilt, anger, denial, and burnout (Harris, 1983). the parent's individual self-concept appears to be an area of particular vulnerability. Depending upon their expectations, the opportunities of living a fuller life through their child are often curtailed or may appear to have been dramatically ended (A Murphy, 1982). Some studies report that mothers commonly report more problems and involvement in these areas than fathers do (Tavormina et al., 1981). However, with more families in which both parents have careers and with fathers in an increasing numbers of families becoming primary caregivers, this situation may be changing.

An excellent source of information and support for parents of a newborn with disabilities is other parents who have shared a similar experience. These more experienced parents can offer insights into services and situations that can be immensely helpful. A hospital social worker or organizations such as Pilot Parents, the Easter Seal Society, and the Association of Retarded Citizens (ARC), can provide new parents with information about how to contact these helping parents.

The Physical Health of a Down Syndrome Child

The birth of a child with Down syndrome may mean not only the birth of a child with significant developmental disabilities, but also the birth of a child with significant medical problems, some of them life-threatening. The medical problems of the child with Down syndrome are multiple and have been outlined in Chapter 1 and subsequent chapters. The presence of any serious medical problems may be a source of great emotional, physical, and financial strains upon the family. When the demands of caretaking become too great, free time becomes nonexistent and "burnout" may set in.

A source of frequent frustration for parents can be finding professional services for their child (Harris, 1983). Locating a pediatrician, neurologist, ophthalmologist, or audiologist who understands the special needs of the child with Down syndrome takes time and can be difficult. Even in urban areas where there is a concentration of services, this may not be easy. Organized parent groups, regional centers, developmental centers, and Down syndrome programs are helpful sources for parents of information about professionals who have special expertise.

Communicating with professionals may also be difficult for parents, particularly at first when they are also attempting to deal with their emotional response to learning that their child has a serious disability. Parents should be encouraged to ask questions and to keep asking until they understand the answers. They should make a list of questions and bring it with them to appointments. Parents should talk openly about their feelings, concerns, and frustrations, to promote an honest and open exchange of information (Hely & Lewis-Beck, 1988). Because parents often find meetings with professionals to be both stressful and intimidating, it is often helpful to use a tape recorder to record meetings with professionals so that they can review what they learn later in a less stressful setting.

Finances and Medical Insurance

The presence of heart disease or other problems may require surgery, hospitalizations, and frequent medical follow-up, all of which are costly. If a child with Down syndrome is not covered by medical insurance at birth, finding insurance coverage may be exceedingly difficult. Parents need to understand their insurance coverage—what services are covered; deductibles, and lifetime-maximum limits; necessity for second opinions; coverage for outpatient services; and so forth. They should be encouraged to keep careful records of all bills for care, prescriptions, and equipment. Often it is helpful if they establish one contact person at the insurance company with whom they can work on a continuing basis (Healy & Lewis-Beck, 1988).

Families of a child with Down syndrome commonly report an inability to leave a job situation simply because insurance coverage on a child would be lost and could not be reestablished in a new job situation. Other parents report seeking employment with large corporations that provide blanket coverage regardless of preexisting medical conditions of members of the family. Even when covered by medical insurance, parents may often accumulate substantial legal expenses in their efforts to ensure that adequate medical coverage is provided for their child. Parent groups have become active in providing education in the areas of finances, income taxes, long-term financial planning, and medical insurance (Harris, 1983).

Other sources of financial assistance may be available through federal or state disability programs. Some of these programs include Medicaid (Title XIX), supplemental security income (SSI) benefits, the medically needy program, and vocational rehabilitation services. Parents' groups are often a good source of information about these programs (Healy & Lewis-Beck, 1988).

Religious Involvement

In some families, religious involvement is a strong positive factor in adjustment. In such instances, when asked about their religious affiliation, the family may describe a deep involvement with their church, often of a "fundamentalist" denomination. As parents, they feel that they are doing for their special child what is expected of them, and do not seem to ask the question that other parents may ask: "Why me?" Religious clergy for these families often provide a strong, ongoing source of support.

Martial Issues

Couples have reported changes in their marriages, including both more intense feelings of intimacy and more tensions, following the birth of a child with disabilities. To a couple with significant martial problems, the birth of a Down syndrome child can be a significant negative factor (Waisbren, 1980). Harris (1983) found that for the mother, an important predictor of her ability to cope with the birth of a child with a disability is the security of the marriage. Parents sometimes report feelings about their child that suggest hopelessness, anger, or rejection. These feelings can cause the relationship between the parents and the child to deteriorate rapidly (Waisbren, 1980). A need to lay blame or to find a cause, often cultural or social, adds additional stress to the marital situation. Fatigue, burnout, and lack of privacy, may accelerate the deterioration of an already-unsound marital relationship, and can disrupt the sexual relationship as well (Harris, 1983). In addition, some parents who have given birth to a child with Down syndrome are concerned about the possibility of having another Down syndrome child. For them, genetic counseling and amniocentesis can provide helpful information. Marriage therapy and counseling may be needed to provide adequate security and communication for a supportive relationship.

Acceptance by Siblings, Extended Family Members, and Others

If the family of the child with Down syndrome has a supportive family and a network of friends, adjustment is facilitated (A. Murphy, 1982). Parents are emotionally vulnerable in the first few months after the birth of a Down syndrome child, and are frequently hypersensitive to the reaction of others

(A. Murphy, 1982). Negative responses from grandparents or extended family members have the potential to be destructive. On the other hand, positive responses from extended family and grandparents can be a great source of emotional support (Harris, 1983).

Grandparents also need to deal with their own feelings about the birth of a grandchild with Down syndrome. In some instances, multigenerational therapy becomes necessary, particularly if extended family members are primary care providers (Harris, 1983).

Siblings are also affected by the birth of a brother or sister with Down syndrome. Sibling emotions may include fear of the disability, shame or guilt, or a feeling of special obligation toward their new brother or sister (Harris, 1983). If the Down syndrome child has multiple problems, siblings may be denied a significant share of parental attention (Harris, 1983). The use of respite care or a babysitter is a necessity if the parents are to have appropriate quality time with all of their children.

Friends can be a source of support for siblings, grandparents, and parents. They can offer to provide respite care, transportation, or just emotional support. Their positive responses are an important source of reassurance for new parents of a child with disabilities. However, the actions of friends can also be detrimental. Those individuals who make inappropriate comments, or who demonstrate fear or a negative feeling of response, can undermine parental morale. Parents often benefit from talking in a parent group about strategies dealing with these often difficult situtations. Role-playing can provide a useful way to practice responses to such situations (Harris, 1983).

Burnout

Many parents of children with Down syndrome believe that if they work hard enough and provide that "little extra" their child will function at a "higher" level of competence (see Table 17.2). One parent explains, "How much is enough! I feel that I should be wearing a chauffeur's hat. I take my daughter to

TABLE 17.1. Factors affecting parents of children with Down syndrome.

No	No	Question
—	—	1. Health of child
—	—	2. Medical insurance coverage
—	—	3. Acceptance of child by family, extended family, and friends
—	—	4. The presence of supportive friends and extended family
—	—	5. Church affiliation
—	—	6. Participation in support groups
—	—	7. Guilt and blame
—	—	8. Health of marriage

TABLE 17.2. Questions commonly asked by parents of children with Down syndrome.

Questions
1. How much intervention is enough?
2. Does early intervention make a major difference?
3. What will really help my child?
4. When will we have reached the point of diminishing returns for our time and effort
5. What are the needs of other family members?
6. Am I being fair to my spouse?
7. Am I jeopardizing our marriage?
8. Am I burning myself out?
9. Am I saving some time just for myself?

preschool three days a week. I drive her to see her speech therapist for one or two hours per week, and physical therapist twice a week. We have her enrolled in a baby swimming program. It seems that almost every week we have an appointment with some specialist. It is not just the driving, we work on exercise at home to overcome her hypotonicity and on recognizing shapes and colors. With the needs of two other children, I never seem to get enough sleep." When asked when she and her husband had last gone out to dinner, she talked about wishing for more time to work on her daughter's language development. Under such conditions some parents begin to burnout (Harris 1983). The burnout phenomenon is accentuated by the fact that over time, as a developmentally disabled child plateaus, or reaches his or her highest level of functioning, progress slows. The parental optimism, once high, begins to diminish as parents become increasingly aware of the youngsters limitations (Harris, 1983). It is important that this phenomenon is recognized by professionals and parent groups that can provide a support network for the parents.

Behavior Management

For some parents, managing a child's behavior is a significant problem. Some parents feel guilty about instituting behavior management techniques for a child with chronic and severe medical problems. Parents may need professional counseling to work through these feelings.

Behavior intervention begins early with the Down syndrome child and is usually a part of the development program offered by schools, regional centers, developmental centers, and behavior management therapy. But if parents do not ask how they should teach their child good behavior until he or she is 14 years old, it is likely that there will already be significant problems. While manipulative behavior may be "cute" in a toddler, it is socially unacceptable in an older child. Behavior management needs are an important issue early in the child's life. Psychologists and educators need to thoroughly convince parents that it is daily living and behavioral skills, not academic skills, that often have the most important impact upon the future of the child with Down syndrome.

Parent Support Groups

Parent groups were first formed in the 1950s when the parents of individuals with a variety of disabilities organized in response to their frustration with professionals and their need for support in coping with the daily concerns of caring for a child with Down syndrome (Perske, 1987). As parent groups evolved, they addressed concerns about education, organization and lobbying, and the development of public policy for persons who are developmentally disabled. In their evolution, local parent groups chartered national organizations such as the National Down Syndrome Congress, the National Association for Retarded Citizens (ARC), and the National Epilepsy Foundation.

A variety of parent support groups exist today. Some are primarily therapy groups in which skilled clinicians supervise therapy. Some groups are exclusively for parents; other groups consist of parents in combination with representatives from many professional disciplines. Groups may provide training, education, or a setting that encourages a small group of parents to share their feelings on a more personal basis (Harris, 1983).

Parent groups can be found in most areas of the United States, but are more concentrated in metropolitan areas. They can be contacted in states through regional medical centers, state departments of human services, primary care providers, developmental centers, or by requesting written information from sponsoring organizations such as Pilot Parents, the National Down Syndrome Congress, or the Association for Retarded Citizens (ARC).

The initial function of most groups is to educate and support parents. As the process continues, the roles often change and the group becomes both a receiver and a provider of information, encouragement, and support to other families.

Nancy Hall, chairperson of the Los Angeles Down Syndrome Parent Group, Inc., explains the benefits of parent support groups:

1. education of parents concerning problems and facts related to Down syndrome;
2. assistance to parents so that they can stay abreast of new developments in the area of developmental disabilities;
3. parental support of each other and sharing of feelings, concerns, and solutions;
4. development of friendships with parents with similar concerns;
5. development of friendships among individuals with Down syndrome;

6. development of core groups that can affect change regarding needs of schools, regional centers, and developmental centres;
7. sharing information about resources and services;
8. counseling for new parents;
9. dissemination of information about Down syndrome to the community;
10. involvement in issues pertaining to advocacy and legislation;
11. cooperation with support groups and agencies concerning disability issues; and
12. organization and provision of social activities for families.

Parents do not need to find a group that is specifically concerned with children with Down syndrome. Just talking to other parents, regardless of the children's particular disabilities, can help new parents realize they are not alone in their concerns. Parents should be reminded, as well, that they can choose the level of their involvement. They may want to attend every meeting, or they may just want to be put on the group's mailing list so that they get the monthly newsletter (Healey & Lewis-Beck, 1988).

Parent support groups can be an important resource for parents of children with Down syndrome. The evolution of the public understanding of Down syndrome and the breaking down of old stereotypes and misinformation are largely the results of the work done by parent groups, which have led the way in educating the public, educators, and professionals. These groups have laid to rest many of the former misunderstandings, confusions, fears, and assumptions surrounding the individual with this syndrome.

A Parent's Perspective

After dealing with the disbelief, anger, and the depression that surround the initial diagnosis of the child with Down syndrome, parents suddenly realize that they have many questions. In fact, it often seems that the more questions they ask, the more questions they have. Some of the questions may arise because the parents cannot accept what they are told; other questions remain because professionals too often use clinical jargon rather than lay terms.

The goals of the parents of a Down syndrome child, like the parents of any child, are for their child to live a happy, productive life; to function in an environment that is appropriate; and to live as independently as possible. However, parents must realize that families are an interactive system (Turnbull & Summers, 1987). In the family with a Down syndrome child, great stresses are exerted on that interactive system. If the system is to function, communication, understanding, and support must be present.

In parenting a child with Down syndrome the major goal is to provide the love, support, understanding, and discipline that all children need. A knowledge of child development is not intuitive, it is learned. With a Down syndrome child, one must be constantly aware of his or her development and be ready to help that child toward the next step.

Parents are their children's most effective advocates. As citizens of the United States, members of these families have the same basic rights as any other citizen. But children with disabilities are also guaranteed additional rights through federal law. Two laws in particular are important for parents of young children with Down syndrome: Public Law 94:142 and Public Law 99:457. P.L. 94:142 states that children with disabilities have a right to a free, appropriate public education. P.L. 99:457 mandates certain preschool and early-intervention services. Under these laws, a child with a developmental disability such as Down syndrome is guaranteed:

- A careful evaluation of his or her strengths and needs.
- Services—educational, residential, vocational, and habilitation—to meet these needs.
- An individualized plan that explains how these needs will be met.
- Help in getting the state and federal assistance—social security, medical care, and vocational services—that are needed.
- Safeguards to the child's rights in the areas of guardianship, least restrictive environment, employment and housing, privacy and confidentiality, credit and insurance, and abuse or neglect (Healy & Lewis-Beck, 1988).

Laws and regulations often seem complex to parents of children with disabilities. If problems arise, parents can contact their state's protection and advocacy office, and agency created by federal law to protect the rights of persons with disabilities.

Finally, parents must keep in mind that their child will some day be an adult, possibly living and working away from home. Planning for their child's adult life should be a goal for parents, and such planning should begin before the child is in high school (Canning, 1987).

With improved educational programs and expanded vocational and residential services, the child with Down syndrome has many more options for an independent and productive life than was possible even a decade ago. Competitive employment and independent or semi-independent living are a reality for many adults with this syndrome. Parents need to be aware of the options available and to advocate for their child so that he or she may reach his or her fullest potential.

Summary

With the birth of a Down syndrome child, a family must address a number of unexpected issues. At present there is no single behavioral or psychological instrument able to analytically measure or evaluate these family issues. It is important that families recognize that there are potential problems areas that, with anticipatory guidance, can be avoided, such as parent support groups, interested professionals, and/or regional health centers and education and vocational programs. Parents of child with Down syndrome should make every effort to be aware of all available options for support for themselves and their child.

References

Burden, R.L. (1980). Measuring the effects of stress on the mothers of handicaped infants: Must depression always follow? *Child Care, Health and Development, 6,* 111–125

Canning, C.D. (1987). A mother's perspective. In S.M. Pueschel, C., Tingey, J.E. Rynders, A.C. Crocker, & D.M. Crutcher (Eds.), *New perspective in Down syndrome* (pp. 307–309). Baltimore, MD: Brookes.

Cobb, L.S., & Hancock, K.A. (1984). Development of the child with a physical disability. *Advances in development and behavioral pediatrics* (pp. 75–107). New York: JAI Press, Inc.

Harris, S.L. (1983). *Families of the developmentally disabled: A guide to behavioral interventions* (pp. 91–92). New York: Pergamon Press.

Healy, A., & Lewis-Beck, J.A. (1988). *The Iowa health care guidelines project: Guidelines for families* (pp. 4–29). Iowa City: Iowa University Affiliated Program.

Murphy, A. (1982). Positive and supportive counseling of parents of infants with Down syndrome. In S.M. Pueschel & J.E. Rynders (Eds.), *Down syndrome, advances in biomedicine and the behavioral science* (pp. 305–330).

Murphy, A. (1982). The family with a handicapped child: A review of the literature. *Development and Behavioral Pediatrics, 3* (2), 73–82.

Murphy, A. (1984). Social service evaluations. In S.M. Pueschel (Eds.), *The young child with Down syndrome* (pp. 87–103). New York: Human Science Press, Inc.

Perske, R. (1987). Attitudes, acceptance, and awareness. In S.M. Pueschel, C. Tingey, J.E. Rynders, A.C. Crocker, & D.M. Crutcher (Eds.), *New perspectives in Down syndrome* (pp. 273–287). Baltimore, MD: Brookes Publishers.

Tavormina, J.B., Boll, T.J., Dunn, N.J., Nuscomb, R.L., & Taylor, J.R. (1981). Psychological effects on parents of raising a physically handicapped child. *Journal of Abnormal Child Psychology, 9* (1), 121–131.

Turnbull, A.P., & Summers, J.A. (1987). From parent involvement to family support: Evolution or revolution. In S.M. Pueschel, C. Tingey, J.E. Rynders, A.C. Crocker, & D.M. Crutcher (Eds.), *New perspectives on Down syndrome* (pp. 289–305). Baltimore, MD: Brookes Publishers.

Waisbren, S.E. (1980). Parents' reactions after the birth of a developmentally disabled child. *American Journal of Mental Deficiency, 84* (4), 345–351.

18
Sexuality, Reproduction, and Contraception

DON C. VAN DYKE AND SUSAN VAN DUYNE

Introduction

It is surprising that in this time of "sexual enlightenment" little has been written addressing sexual issues as related to individuals with mental retardation. In spite of the fact that individuals with Down syndrome are healthier, have a longer life expectancy, and are no longer residing in institutions, the literature on sexuality and contraception is small. In spite of the fact that sexuality is an area of major concern for parents of children with Down syndrome, there is surprisingly little in the literature discussing its importance.

Individuals with Down syndrome continue to be burdened with the stigma associated with sexuality in persons who are mentally retarded. Though our present era of sexual enlightenment acknowledges that sexual expression is appropriate, the exceptions to this attitude lag far behind for those who are mentally compromised. In fact, while mating, marrying, and having children is the normal sexual model, when a person with Down syndrome expresses or acts out these same desires, such behavior is commonly perceived as inappropriate. In investigations by Pueschel who measured parental perceptions of social interactions, interest in the opposite sex, and sexual functioning in the individual with Down syndrome, it was found that at least 50% of these individuals showed interest in the opposite sex and were attending social gatherings (Pueschel et al., 1987). Thus, the interest is there; how society will respond to this interest is an unanswered question.

Sexuality

Pueschel and Rynders (1982) presented a survey in the literature pointing out that what is written tends to be descriptive rather than "constructive." They examined the views expressed by Wolfensberger (1972) regarding the criteria for heterosexual relationships among mentally retarded adults. The criteria for heterosexual relationships among people who were mentally retarded was no more stringent than that of other heterôsexuals. Discussing the belief that human sexual expression necessitates "responsible" behavior, however, Wolfensberger failed to address the cognitive dissonance that continues to exist in our society.

Parents of children with Down syndrome, like all parents, are concerned about sexual education, dating, and related issues. Many parents have expressed concerns about teaching their children appropriate means of expressing affection. Adolescents with Down syndrome are often observed to be too physical when they demonstrate affection, so that sometimes their actions are seen as "unacceptable" in our society.

Another frequently expressed parental concern is the fear their children may be sexually abused. In a study by Chamberlain, Rauth, Passer, McGrath, and Burket (1984), it was demonstrated that mildly retarded children are at the greatest risk for sexual abuse, whereas children with severe retardation may be at a lower risk than those with normal intelligence. Thus, the Down syndrome child who normally falls in the mild to moderate range of mental retardation is, statistically, a potential target for sexual abuse. Parents often relate, "I think Johnny [or Betty] would go off with anyone who was nice to him [or her]." In questioning on the Vineland, the answers tend commonly to be positive when the parents are asked whether their child demonstrates understanding that it is unsafe to accept rides, food, or money from strangers. Few parents of children with Down syndrome express confidence, however, in their child's response to such questions. Their underlying problem with this area of questioning is that it is difficult for individuals with Down syndrome to generalize in the formation of concepts. These individuals can be taught responsible behavior. They can be taught not to accept candy. They cannot, however, always be taught not to accept rides from strangers. The problem arises when the situation deviates from the script that they have learned.

In addition, some individuals view mentally retarded individuals as oversexed and sexually irresponsible. Others view them as totally lacking any sex drive at all. Pueschel noted that many youngsters with Down syndrome had expressed a desire to marry, but only a few had an interest in sexual relationship (Pueschel et al., 1987). Studies have indicated that individuals with lower IQs have shown delayed sexual maturation and lack sexual drive. However, it has also been demonstrated that mentally retarded individuals functioning in the mild to moderate range do demonstrate a real sexual awareness (Chamberlain et al., 1984).

Reproduction and Contraception

Sex education, sterilization, and contraceptives are major concerns expressed by parents of children with Down syndrome. Parents of daughters with Down syndrome demonstrate the highest level of concern and anxiety.

In regard to sexual maturation in Down syndrome, studies show that the average onset of menstruation in females is 12 years 6 months, with regular menstrual cycles. A study by Scola and Pueschel in 1985 showed that most do not require help with menstrual hygiene (Pueschel et al., 1987). Studies of ovulatory patterns of females with Down syndrome by Tricomi, Valenti, and Hall (1964) showed that only 31% showed no evidence of ovulation. Reports from the literature clearly document the fact that females with Down syndrome can become pregnant, delivering both normal and Down syndrome children (Jagiello, 1981).

Males with Down syndrome are sterile. The frequency of hypospadias and cryptorchidism is equal to that of the general population (Hsiang et al., 1987). In the male with Down syndrome, penile length and testicular volume have been shown to be significantly below the norm, with serum FSH and LH levels significantly elevated above the mean. It is felt that primary gonadel deficiency is common in Down syndrome males and is progressive from birth to adolescence (Hsiang et al., 1987).

Sex education has become a major area of both concern and controversy in educational system for both disabled and nondisabled individuals. For the most part, the educational system now includes sex education classes as part of its curriculum. However, when it comes to such curricula for developmentally or physically handicapped individuals, most educational systems are afraid to address the sexual education issue and wish to avoid the contraceptive issue with the developmentally delayed populations. Parents who push school officials for such instruction or ask questions regarding sex education and contraception are usually referred to a physician, most often a specialist in obstetrics-gynecology who has had little experience with adolescent gynecology and no experience with persons who are developmentally disabled. The results are often unsatisfactory for all parties concerned. Most parents do not seek out further consultation from the medical community or ask additional questions of the school system. This is unfortunate, because adolescent females with Down syndrome are not provided with the necessary gynecological care received by females without Down syndrome. In working with clinics that serve the adolescent female with Down syndrome, it is a frequent observation that these individuals rarely or never have a breast exam, an internal gynecological exam, or a PAP-test—routine medical procedures for the developmentally normal female population.

The issue of contraception generates enormous controversy. There are special needs for fertility control by adolescents who are mentally retarded. Each case must be assessed individually, in hopes of finding a favorable balance between safety and effectiveness. Injectable medroxyprogesterone acetate (DMPA) is a progestogen that has been used for contraception; it has not, however, been approved by the FDA because of the unresolved question regarding its potential carcinogenicity. IUDs have been advocated, with caution, for developmentally delayed individuals. However, they carry with them significant problems, including increased expulsion rate of the IUD and pelvic infections. Continuation rates for oral contraceptives have not been high. The decision to use oral contraceptives often implies the presence of an adult who is motivated to supervise their administration (Chamberlain et al., 1984).

Sterilization is a multifaceted and controversial issue for parents (Passer, Rauch, Chamberlain, McGrath, Burket, 1984). A common reason given by parents seeking sterilization of their mentally retarded daughter is protection from pregnancy. Sterilization will accomplish birth control and may resolve the problems of menstrual hygiene, but it does little toward addressing the other areas of sexuality. In many states, there is no statute that permits sterilization of mentally retarded individuals.

Only recently has society begun to recognize that citizens with mental retardation should have the same rights as those with normal intelligence (Kindred et al., 1976). Two extreme positions are held by those opposed to involuntary sterilization. One argues that the right to bear a child cannot be taken away by anyone; the other, that the right *not* to bear children is a compelling social issue (Vining & Freedman, 1978). In a study by Passer et al. (1984), 85% of parents with children who were mentally retarded favored some form of statute permitting sterilization. Most seem to be searching for a moderate position that would permit the procedure under certain circumstances and with specific safeguards, checks, and balances (Passer et al., 1984).

In summary, the most commonly asked questions by parents of children with Down syndrome are:

1. What are the sexual needs of the Down syndrome child, female and male?
2. What do parents of adolescent and adult individuals (both female and male) with Down syndrome feel is appropriate and acceptable sexual behavior?
3. What means of sexual education for females and males with Down syndrome are effective and supportive?
4. Is sterilization appropriate/and or available in some instances? Are appropriate contraceptive methods available and where can they be obtained?

Summary

The issues of sexual activity, sexual abuse, contraception, and sex education for persons with Down syndrome are similar to the issues that face other disability populations. The sexual needs of these individuals should be discussed and understood at home, at school, and by the public as a whole. Efforts may be necessary to facilitate patient/parent communication and comprehension—difficulties that often pose substantial barriers to the acquisition of needed services. The network of developmental disabilities and diagnostic programs that exist in some states and regional centers, such as those in the state of California, need to push for comprehensive adolescent health care, including gynecological services and family planning. Regional settings offer a unique opportunity to better understand and meet the contraceptive and obstetrical-gynecological needs of the persons who are developmentally delayed.

Many parents believe that the greatest risk of sexual assault is to the severely retarded female; however, studies have demonstrated that it is the mildly to moderately mentally retarded female who is at the greatest risk. Developmental disability programs need to make a special issue of addressing the potential problems of sexual abuse in this population.

The issue of sterilization continues to be controversial. It is felt that this issue needs to be addressed on the public level, with increasing efforts made for modernization of sterilization laws in all states. It is felt that ongoing study is needed in order to understand the views of patients and their families.

References

Chamberlain, A., Rauth, J., Passer, A., McGrath, M., & Burket, R. (1984). Issues in fertility control for mentally retarded female adolescents: 1. Sexual activity, sexual abuse and contraception. *Pediatrics, 73* (4), 445–450.

Hsiang, Y.H., Berkovitz, G.D., Bland, G.L., Migeon, C.J., & Warren, A.C. (1987). Gonadal function in patients with Down syndrome. *American Journal of Medical Genetics, 27* (2), 449–458.

Jagiello, G. (1981). Reproduction in Down syndrome. In F. de la Cruz, & P.S. Gerald (Eds.), *Down syndrome research perspectives* (pp. 151–162). Baltimore, MD: University Park Press.

Kindred, M., et al. (Eds.). (1976). *The mentally retarded citizen and the law*. New York: MacMillan Publishing.

Passer, A., Rauh, J., Chamberlain, A., McGrath, M., & Burket, R. (1984). Issues in fertility control for mentally retarded female adolescents: 2. Parental attitudes towards sterilization. *Pediatrics, 73* (4), 451–454.

Pueschel, S.M., & Rynders, J.E. (1982). *Down's syndrome: Advances in bio-medicine and behavioral science*. Cambridge MA: Ware Press.

Pueschel, S.M., Tingey, C., Rynders, J.E., Crocker, A.C., & Crutcher, D.M. (1987). *New Perspectives on Down syndrome*. Baltimore, MD: Paul H. Brookes Publishing Co.

Tricomi, V., Valenti, C., & Hall, J.E. (1964). Ovulatory patterns in Down's syndrome. *American Journal of Obstetrics and Gynecology, 89*, 651–656.

Vining, E.P.G., & Freeman, J.M. (1978). Sterilization and the retarded female: Is advocacy depriving patients of their rights? *Pediartrics, 62* (5), 850–852.

Wolfensberger, W. (1972). *Normalization: The principle of normalization in human services*. Toronto: National Institute of Mental Retardation.

19
Alternative and Controversial Therapies

DON C. VAN DYKE, SUSAN VAN DUYNE, OARIONA LOWE, AND FRANCES HEIDE

Introduction

"Your child has Down syndrome," is, for many parents, the start of a long search for knowledge, guidance, and support that will improve the quality of life for their child. Over time, this search often leads them to a variety of intervention programs, some of which are termed "alternative therapies." Too often, standard medical practice offers parents little information regarding the etiology of this syndrome, and, for some parents, the frustration that follows becomes a driving force in their efforts to obtain a solution to the medical and development problems of their child.

Some alternative therapies that are offered to parents of children with Down syndrome are, "in terms of modern biological and medical knowledge, controversial" (Golden, 1984, 1987). These therapies are often based on the use of dietary supplements, physical therapy treatments, or injections of "natural materials" (Horrobin & Pueschel, 1982). In a review of the case histories of 190 individuals with Down syndrome presented in the introduction and appendix 1, 21 of the 190 (or 11%) had received cell therapy (Van Dyke et al., 1989). When questioned about megavitamin therapy, 36 of the 190 (or 19%) had received this type of therapy. It would appear from this sample that alternative therapies are used with a significant number of infants and children with Down syndrome.

Review of Therapies

Thyroid Hormone

The administration of thyroid hormone extract, one of the first therapies for Down syndrome was introduced by T.T. Smith in 1896. Over the years a number of physicians, including Benda (1960), advocated its use. Studies by Koch, Share, and Gralicker (1965) did not find significant differences between individuals with Down syndrome who were treated with thyroid and others who were untreated. However, the incidence of thyroid dysfunction, particularly hypothyroidism secondary to Hashimoto's thyroiditis, has been documented as increasing with age in Down syndrome individuals, with a reported incidence as high as 30% (Pueschel & Pezzullo, 1985). It would seem evident that Down syndrome individuals with hypothyroid disease benefit significantly from thyroid replacement therapy.

Cell Therapy

Cell therapy, or sicca cell or dry cell therapy, has been used since the 1930s, beginning with Dr. Paul Niehans (Schmid, 1983). This controversial alternative therapy injects freeze-dried cells from the organs of fetal sheep, cows, and/or rabbits. The major proponent of this therapy in the last 20 years has been Dr. Franz Schmid (1983). According to Schmid, injected fetal cells activated brain growth because of a suppressive affinity between the cells of a particular organ from the embryonic animal and/or the compromised organ, causing the "revitalized" cell to become the nucleus for tissue regeneration (Schmid, 1976).

Cell therapy is usually only a part of the regimen that individuals use in alternative therapy programs. Such programs often consist of cell therapy injections, speech therapy, sound framing, physical therapy, "pedagogy measures," vitamin prescriptions, minerals, and tryptophan (Schmid, 1976). The individual treatment plan varies from child to child based on preceived needs as determined by the physician. According to Schmid, cell therapies result in an IQ increase, improvement in speech, improved motor and social abilities, increased height, and increased head circumference and brain size (Schmid, 1976). A double-blind study by Black, Kato, and Walker (1966) found no evidence that sicca cell treatment improved children's development. Other investigators have not found any significant difference between experimental and control groups (Bardon, 1964; Share, 1976). German investigators, including Bremer (1975) and Schulte (1975) found no evidence that sicca cell injections were effective in ameliorating the symptoms of Down syndrome.

In a study of 1220 children over a period of 1 to 20 years, Schmid and others administered to 867+ subjects two to three series of implantations at five-month periods (Preus & Fewell, 1983). Many parents take their children to Europe for treatments, commenting, "what do we have to lose?" However, other parents feel differently. Karp (1983) questioned this perspective because of the potential for biological side-effects, as well as the issue of cost. In addition, there have been some concerns regarding anaphylactic reactions to cell therapy injections, as well as more recent concerns regarding the potential for fatal transmission of a slow virus infection. This is particularly cogent in light of the recent demonstration of progressive degenerative CNS disease seen in several individuals receiving growth hormone derived from human cadavers. Use of cell therapy in the United States has not been approved by the Food and Drug Administration or the American Medical Association (Karp, 1983).

Orthomolecular Therapy

Orthomolecular therapy is defined by Dr. Linus Pauling as "the treatment of mental disorders by the provision of the optimum molecular environment for the mind; especially optimum concentrations of substances normally found in the human body" (Turkel, 1963). This approach in the treatment of Down syndrome emphasizes the numerous physiological dysfunctions in identified "serum nutritional deficiencies" associated with this syndrome (Turkel, 1963).

Since 1940, Turkel (1975) has been major proponents of the "U" series as a means of ameliorating Down syndrome. The "U" series contains over 50 substances which Turkel claims stimulate a child's metabolism and eliminate waste products. Anecdotal reports of successes describe marked improvement in children treated with this therapy, including "straightening of the first finger, regression of premature aging, improvement in IQ, and improvement of aesthetic appearances" (Turkel, 1975). Studies by White and Kaplitz (1964) did not find any significant improvement with vitamin therapy. Studies by Bumbalo (1964), specifically of the "U" series using a double-blind study, found no improvement except in socialization.

Interest in vitamin therapy was recently regenerated when Harrell et al. (1981) reported that the IQ scores of a group of mentally retarded children had improved following the administration of megavitamins and minerals. The children who showed the most improvement were children with Down syndrome. Following publication of the study results, many parents and physicians began using the Harrell regimen. Later replication of the Harrell study did not support the preliminary results (Golden, 1984; 1987). Continuing concerns have been raised about the efficacy and expense of megavitamin and mineral approaches and the issue of safety, particularly with the fat-soluble vitamins such as vitamin A (Golden, 1987).

Dimethyl Sulfoxide

The use of dimethyl sulfoxide (DMSO) for treatment of Down syndrome began following a report by Aspillage, Morizon, and Vendano (1975) that claimed an improvement in intellectual functioning as a result of its administration. Questions raised about the design of the study resulted in a second short-term study to determine the efficacy of the use of DMSO. This study did not demonstrate significant improvements in the academic or behavioral areas of either children with Down syndrome or other children with mental retardation (Gabourie, Becker, & Bateman, 1975).

Other Compounds

Other compounds have been suggested as treatment for Down syndrome, including glutamic acid and its derivatives, (Gadson, 1951), dehydro-epiandrosterone (DeMoragas, 1958), pituitary extract (Benda, 1960), 5-hydro-xytrytophan (Pueschel, 1980), and serotonin (Coleman 1973; Tu, 1965). In follow-up studies, none of these compounds has been proven to significantly ameliorate the symptoms of Down syndrome.

Other Therapy Programs

Therapy programs, particularly early intervention, are frequently offered to children with Down syndrome. A questionnaire given to parents or caregivers of the 190 individuals in this study, showed that 64% of their children with Down syndrome had received or were receiving speech therapy, 56% physical therapy, and 48% occupational therapy. A smaller number (17%) had received or were receiving some type of resource teaching or tutoring. Many communities refer all developmentally disabled children or children at risk for developmental disability to an intervention program. Home- and center-based neurodevelopmental therapy is common in most urban areas. parents of children with Down syndrome are frequently trained in behavior-modification techniques. Recent studies suggest that children with down syndrome can benefit from training in specific areas provided by these programs (Harris, 1981). Other studies done to evaluate these programs indicate that there are a number of important issues that have not been or are only currently being addressed.

Patterning Therapy

Patterning has not been specifically studied or claimed as a therapeutic method for treatment of Down syndrome, although an unspecific number of children are receiving this therapy and some professionals have strongly promoted such programs. In a matched control study, Sparrow and Zigler (1978) showed that while all the children who received this type of therapy showed some improvement in performance, no intergroup differences were observed. While Sparrow and Zigler's findings imply that treatment and nontreatment groups did just as well, the results are disputed by some professionals who strongly support patterning as an alternative therapy.

Craniofacial, Orthodontic, and Plastic Surgery

The face of a person with Down syndrome is characterized by flatness and small, centrally placed features. The flatness is accentuated by the broad, flat nose. Carter and McCarthy (1951) described the face in the newborn as being centrally depressed, with chubby cheeks emphasizing the flat appearance. Reporting on the facial characteristics of Down syndrome, Chicoine (1962) suggested that the facial appearance in this syndrome is so general and typical that diagnosis could be based on this alone. He found the head small for the child's age; the tongue protruding; and the nose short, broadened and flattened.

The craniofacial structures of Down syndrome individuals is characterized as brachycephalia, flat-bridged nose, delayed closure of sutures, slanting orbits, epicanthal folds, underdeveloped midface, prominent mandible with increased gonial angle, and frequent absence of a frontal sinus. Some other craniofacial anomalies observed are small mouth, constricted facial features, macroglossia, and fissured tongue. The palate has been designated as one of the nine primary sites of developmental retardation; it is observed that the palatal vaults are narrow and shorter than normal palates. The facial profile is flat with a short nose. The dental disharmonies of malocclusion are characterized by mesiocclusion with anterior crossbite and constriction of the dental arches. While there is a significant deficiency in the gross area of the midface, mandible, and endocranium, the magnitude of the midface deficiency becomes progressively greater with age in relation to both gross area and endocranium. Conversely, the magnitude of mandibular deficiency remains constant with age in the same relationships.

The choices of treatments for the correction of the midface and relative mandibular prognathism often found with Down syndrome may be surgical or orthodontic. Often these maxillo-mandibular deformities have been treated by anterior surgical repositioning of the maxilla. Orthodontic appliances have been designed, which place an anterior force on the maxilla in order to correct these deformities. Plastic or craniofacial surgery as a remedial approach for individuals with Down syndrome has been an area of considerable interest in the last several years (Lemperle & Radu, 1980). The first to use this approach was Höhler (1977) in Germany, who reduced the long tongue, enlarged the nose and chin, removed the epicanthal folds, and corrected the slant axis of the female with Down syndrome. By 1983, over 280 children had been operated upon in Germany, and 11 in Australia (Rozner, 1983). The most common procedures are tongue reduction, nasal implant, lateral canthopexy, cheek implants, chin implants, and tissue excision, with the first three procedures being the ones most commonly performed. The general goals for craniofacial surgery in the child with Down syndrome has been to lessen the negative consequences of the condition, maximize physical/mental development, modify facial appearance, and improve social prognosis (Feurstein, 1983).

Research into craniofacial surgery in Down syndrome is relatively new. Some studies have been subjective and anecdotal. Strong parental pressure is developing in the United States and other countries to make plastic surgery more readily available. Some of the issues raised by research on plastic surgery in Down syndrome are:

1. Is it appropriate to carry out cosmetic surgery on a child for purely social reasons?

2. Is there sufficient data to determine whether such surgery accomplishes its goals?
3. Who makes the decision regarding plastic surgical correction?
4. What are the complications and morbidity of such procedures?
5. Is the child's sense of self-identity negatively affected by the change in appearance?

A symposium has summarized the effects in regard to objective benefits, changes in patient attractiveness, and changes in social perception (Lefebvine, 1987). Craniofacial surgical procedures in Down syndrome appear to have no effect on the auditory quality of speech, but do improve the visual quality of speech. There are minimal improvements in chewing and biting. Some Down syndrome children had less mouth breathing; others had decreased upper respiratory infections. There were no significant changes in IQ or family function.

Evaluation of patient attractiveness produced a wide spectrum of responses. Down syndrome parents felt that the appearance of their children was improved. The children themselves were not clearly positive or negative, and the responses of objective raters ranged from no change to slightly worse in appearance (Lefebvine, 1987). In regard to social perception, Down syndrome parents described their children as more outgoing, social, and confident. However, school teachers reported such changes in only 30% of children (Lefebvine, 1987). More thorough long-term studies need to be conducted to determine the effects of such procedures on the quality of life for the individual with Down syndrome.

Evaluation of the occlusal disharmony in Down syndrome individuals shows an increased incidence of Class III malocclusion, crossbite, and open bite, and decreased arch length and circumference (Jensen et al., 1973). The magnitude of the midface deficiency become progressively greater with age in relationship to the gross area and endocranium. Orthodontic appliances have been designed to place an anterior force on the maxilla to correct these deformities (Jackson et al., 1979). Appliances designed to treat maxillary hypoplasia may also establish psychological and anatomical functional occlusion, and influence maxillary and mandibular growth patterns by inhibiting and/or redirecting normal growth in children. A modified maxillary protraction face mask (MMPF) and rapid palatal expansion device (RPE) is being used in the correction of midfacial deficiency and relative mandibular prognathism for the non-Down syndrome population. There is increasing interest in using these devices (MMPF/RPE) or their modifications with children who have Down syndrome.

Summary

The realization that the symptoms associated with Down syndrome will be life-long motivates for families and professionals to search for solutions to ameliorate these symptoms. Although the "jury is still out" on some therapies, such as orthodontic therapy and craniofacial surgery, there is no evidence or support for other therapies, such as orthomolecular therapy, thyroid supplementation, and the long list of vitamins and other supplemental therapies when scientific method, analytic and statistical scrutiny have been applied.

There is increasing interest in craniofacial surgery in children with Down syndrome. However, no long-term controlled studies showing the efficacy of such surgery have been completed. The use of orthodontic appliances presents an early means of correction of some of these abnormalities. Hopefully, research will be done to determine which individuals would benefit from such intervention.

The approach should be to involve the presentation of all available information to the child's parents at an appropriate time and in a manner the parents can understand and assimilate. Questions and issues, even controversial ones, should be discussed rather than avoided. Whatever decision the parents make regarding alternative therapies, it is important for the primary service provider to continue to offer the child appropriate medical care, ongoing monitoring, and support and guidance throughout this process to all of the family.

References

Aspillage, M.J., Morizon, G., & Vendano, I.A. (1975). Dimethylsulfoxide therapy in severe retardation in Mongoloid children. *Annals of the New York Academy of Science, 243*, 421–431.

Bardon, L.M. (1964). Sicca cell treatment in Mongolism. *Lancet, 2*, 234–235.

Benda, C.E. (1960). *Child with Mongolism*. New York: Grune and Stratton.

Black, D.B., Kato, J.G., & Walker, G.W. (1966). A study of improvement in mentally retarded children accruing from sicca cell therapy. *American Journal of Mental Deficiencies, 70* (4), 499–508.

Bremmer, J.H. (1975). Discussion of cell therapy in children with relationship to pediatric-metabolic issues. *Mschr Kinderheik, 123*, 674–675.

Bumbalo, T.S. (1964). Negative results: Treatment of Down syndrome with the "U" series. *Journal of the American Medical Association, 361*, 1987.

Carter, C.O., & McCarthy, D. (1951) Incidence of Mongolism and its diagnosis in the newborn. *British Journal of Social Medicine, 5*, 83.

Chicoine, L. (1962). Child deformities. *Canada Nurse, 58*, 1015–1017.

Coleman, M. (Ed.) (1973). *Serotonin in Down's syndrome*. New York: Elsevier Publishers.

DeMoragas, J. (1958). Treatment of Mongolism with dehydroepiandrosterone. *Reviews of Espde Pediatrics, 14*, 545.

Feurstein, R. (1983). Down syndrome surgery: A part of an active modification approach. *Symposium on the future of seriously impaired infants: Where do professionals and society stand?* Annual meeting of the American Orthopsychiatric Association, Boston.

Gabourie, J., Becker, J.W., & Bateman, B. (1975). Oral dimethylsulfoxide in mental retardation. Part I: Preliminary behavioral and psychometric data. In S.W. Jacobs &

R. Herschler (Eds.), *Biological actions of dimethyl sulfoxide, Annals of the NY Academy of Science, 243*, 1–508.

Gadson, E.J. (1951). Glutamic acid and mental deficiency. *American Journal of Mental Deficiency, 55*, 521–528.

Golden, G.S. (1984). Controversies in therapies for children with Down syndrome. *Pediatrics in Review, 6*(4), 116–120.

Golden, G.S. (1987). A hard look at fad therapies for developmental disorders. *Contemporary Pediatrics*, 47–60.

Goldstein, H. (1956). Treatment of congenital acromicria syndrome in children. *Archives of Pediatrics*, 13–153.

Harrell, R.F., Capp, R.H., Davis, D.R., Peerless, J., & Ravitz, L.R. (1981). Can nutritional supplements help mentally retarded children? An exploratory study. *Proceedings of the National Academy of Science USA, 78*(1), 574–578.

Harris, S.R. (1981). Effects of neurodevelopmental therapy on motor performance of infants with Down syndrome. *Developmental Med Child Neurology, 23*, 477–483.

Höhler, H. (1977). Changes in facial expression as a result of plastic surgery in Mongoloid children. *Aesthetic Plastic Surgery, 1*, 225.

Horrobin, J.M., & Pueschel, S.M. (1982). Medical care and management. In S. Pueschel & J. Rynders (Eds.), *Down syndrome: Advances in biomedicine and the behavioral sciences* (pp. 269–303). Cambridge MA: Ware Press.

Jackson, G.W., Kokich, B.G., & Shapiro, P.A. (1979). Experimental and post-experimental response to anteriorly directed extra oral forces in young Macaca Nemestrina. *American Journal of Orthodontics, 75*(3), 318–333.

Jensen, G.M. Cleall, J.F., & Yip, A.F. (1973). Dentoalveolar morphology and developmental changes in Down's syndrome (trisomy 21). *American Journal of Orthodontics, 64*(6), 607–618.

Karp, L.E. (1983). New hope for the retarded? *American Journal of Medical Genetics, 16*(1), 1–5.

Koch, R., Share, J., & Graliker, B.V. (1965). The effects of cytomel on young children with Down's Syndrome (Mongolism): A double-blind longitudinal study. *Journal of Pediatrics, 66*, 776.

Lefebvine, A. (1987). *Should retarded people have surgery? The psychological aspects of craniofacial problems. Surgery is not enough.* Dallas, TX: The International Craniofacial Institute Conference.

Lemperle, G., & Radu, D. (1980). Facial plastic surgery in children with Down's syndrome. *Plastic and Reconstructive Surgery, 66*(3), 337–342.

Preus, J.B., & Fewell, R.R. (1983). Cell therapy and the treatment of Down syndrome: A review of research. *Trisomy 21, 1*(1), 3–8.

Pueschel, S.M., & Pezzullo, J.C. (1985). Thyroid dysfunction in Down syndrome. *American Journal of Diseases of Children, 139*, 636–369.

Pueschel, S.M., Reed, R.B., Cronk, C.E., & Goldstein, B.I. (1980). 5-Hydroxytryptophan and/or pyridoxine. Their effect in young children with Down's syndrome. *American Journal of Diseases of Children, 134*(9), 838–844.

Rozner, L. (1983). Facial plastic surgery for Down's syndrome. *Lancet, 11*(1) 8337, 1320–1323.

Schmid, F. (1976). *Mongolism syndrome.* Deutsch Hebammen-Z, 28, 169–173.

Schmid, F. (1983). *Cell therapy: A new dimension of medicine.* Thun, Switzerland: Ott. Publishers.

Schulte, F.J. (1975). Discussion concerning the treatment of Down syndrome with special reference to cell therapy from a neurophysiologic-neuropediatric point of view. *Mschr Kinderheik, 123*, 671–674.

Share, J.B. (1976). Reviewing of drug treatment for Down's syndrome persons. *American Journal of Mental Deficiencies, 80* (4), 388–393.

Smith, T.T. (1986). A peculiarity in the shape of the hand in idiots of the Mongol type. *Pediatrics, 2*, 315–320.

Sparrow, S, & Zigler, E. (1978). Evaluation of pattern and treatment for retarded children. *Pediatrics, 62* (2), 137–150.

Tu, J.B., & Zellweger, H. (1965). Blood serotonin deficiency in Down' syndrome. *Lancet, 2* (415), 715—716.

Turkel, H. (1963). Medical treatment of Mongolism. *Proceedings: Second International Congress on Mental Retardation, Vienna 1*, 409.

Turkel, H. (1975). Medical amelioration of Down syndrome incorporating the orthomolecular approach. *Journal of Orthomolecular Psychiatry, 41* (2), 102–115.

Van Dyke, D.C., Lang, D.J., van Duyne, S., Chang, H. (1989). Cell Therapy in Down syndrome: A retrospective study. *Pediatrics.*

White, D., & Kaplitz, S.E. (1964). Treatment of down syndrome with a vitamin-mineral hormonal preparation. *International Copenhagen Congress: Scientific Study of Mental Retardation, 1*, 224.

Suggested Reading List

American Academy of Pediatrics, Committee on Sports Medicine. (1984), Atlantoaxial stability in Down syndrome. *Pediatrics, 74*, 152–154.

Carr, J. (1975). *Young children with Down syndrome*. London: Butterworth Publishers.

Cunningham, C. (1982). *Down syndrome: An introduction for parents*. London: Souvenir Press.

de la Cruz, F.F., & Gerald, P.S. (Eds.). (1981). *Trisomy 21 (Down syndrome) research perspectives*. Baltimore, MD: University Park Press.

Diamond, L.S., Lynne, D., & Sigmand, B. (1981). Orthopedic disorders in children with Down syndrome. *Orthopedic Clinics of North America, 12*(1), 57–71.

Gibson, D. (1978). *Down syndrome*. Cambridge: University Press.

Golden, G.S. (1984). Controversies in therapies for children with Down syndrome. *Pediatrics in Review, 6*(4), 116–20.

Greenwood, R.D., & Nadus, A.S. (1976). The clinical course of cardiac disease in Down syndrome. *Pediatrics, 58*(6), 893–897.

Harris, S. (1984). Down syndrome. In S.K. Campbell (Ed.), *Clinics and physical therapy: Pediatric neurologic disorders*. New York: Churchill-Livingston.

Meyers, L. (1989). Using computers to teach children with Down syndrome spoken and written language skills. In Nadel (Ed.), *Psychology of Down Syndrome* (pp. 247–265). Boston: MIT Press.

Miller, M., & Cosgriff, M.J. (1983) Hematologic abnormalities in newborn infants with Down syndrome. *American Journal of Medical Genetics, 16*, 1972–1977.

Morss, J.R. (1983). Cognitive development in the Down syndrome infant: Slow or different? *British Journal of Educational Psychology, 53*, 40–47.

Patterson, D. (1987). The cause of Down syndrome. *Scientific American, 242*(2), 52–57.

Pipes, P.L. & Holm, E.A., (1980). Feeding children with Down syndrome. *Journal of the American Dietic Association, 77*(3), 277–282.

Pueschel, S.M. (1984). *The young child with Down syndrome*. New York: Human Science Press, Inc.

Pueschel, S.M. (1988). Atlantoaxial instability in Down syndrome. *Pediatrics, 81*(6), 879–880.

Pueschel, S.M., & Rynders, J. (1982). *Down syndrome: Advances in biomedicine and behavioral science*. Cambridge, MA: Wehr Press.

Pueschel, S.M., Tingey, C., Rynders, J.E., Crocker, A.C., & Crutcher, D.M. (1987). *New perspectives on Down syndrome*. Baltimore, MD: Paul H. Brookes Publishing Co.

Robinson, L.L. et al. (1984). Down syndrome and acute leukemia in children: A ten-year retrospective study. Children's Cancer Study Group. *Journal of Pediatrics, 195*, 235–242.

Scoggin, C.H. & Patterson, D. (1982). Down's syndrome as a model disease. *Archives of Internal Medicine, 1942* (3), 462–464.

Shapiro, M.V., & France, T.D. (1985). Ocular features of Down syndrome. *American Journal of Ophthalmology, 99*, 650–663.

Smith, G.R., & Berg, J.M. (1976). *Down's anomaly* (2nd ed.). New York: Churchill-Livingston.

Strome, M. (1981). Down syndrome: A modern otorhinolaryngolocal pespective. *Laryngoscope, 91* (1), 1581–1594.

Zellweger, H.U. (1981). The story of Down syndrome which preceded Langdon Down. *Down syndrome, 4* (1), 1–2.

Appendices (1–13)

1. Demographics of Down Syndrome Population

I. Subjects

		N	%
Sex:	Males	91	47.9
	Females	99	52.1
Age distribution (months):	Range: 2–230		
	Mean: 59.41		
	Median: 37.5		
	STD dev.: 56.80		

Hollingshead social class:

	N	%
I	29	15.3
II	35	18.4
III	49	25.8
IV	53	27.9
V	16	8.4
No information	8	4.2

Mean: 2.83 STD dev. 1.33

Siblings of subject population:

Number of siblings	N	%
0	50	26.3
1	66	34.7
2	36	18.9
3	21	11.1
4	7	2.1
5	1	0.5
6	2	1.1
7	4	2.1

8	1	0.5
9	2	1.1

Birth rank:

Birth rank	N	%
No information	6	3.2
1	79	41.6
2	57	30.0
3	21	11.1
4	13	6.8
5	5	2.6
7	3	1.6
8	3	1.6
9	1	0.5
10	2	1.1

Mean: 2.21 STD dev. 1.73

Number of older brothers:
Mean: 0.553 STD dev. 1.00
Range: (0–7)

Number of younger brothers:
Mean: 0.22 STD dev. 0.51
Range: (0–3)

Number of older sisters:
Mean: 0.59 STD dev. 1.05
Range: (0–7)

Number of younger sisters:
Mean: 0.17 STD dev. 0.45
Range: (0–3)

Number of People Living in Home:
Mean: 4.60 STD dev. 1.67
Range: (2–15)

II. Mothers of Down Syndrome Population

Age distribution (years): Range: (18–46)
Mean: 30.26
Median: 28
STD dev.: 5.87

Mother's race:

	N	%
No information	11	5.8
Caucasian	136	71.6
Black	3	1.6
Hispanic	31	16.3
Jewish	7	3.7
Other	1	0.5

Mother's religion:

	N	%
No information	68	35.8
None	21	11.1
Catholic	50	26.3
Protestant	29	15.3
Jewish	8	4.2
Other	14	7.4

Mother's education:

Years	N	%
No information	16	7.84
2	1	0.5
6	1	0.5
9	1	0.5
10	5	2.6
11	3	1.6
12	44	23.2
13	16	8.4
14	31	16.3
15	9	4.7
16	37	19.5
17	7	3.7
18	18	9.5
19	1	0.5
19+	1	0.5

Mean: 13.14 STD dev. 4.82

Mother's occupation:

	N	%
No information	179	94.2
Owner of large firm Higher executive Major professional	2	1.1
Business manager Owner of medium business Lesser professional	2	1.1
Owner of small independent business Administrative personnel Minor professional	2	1.1
Technician/clerical/sales person Owner of very small business	1	0.5

Skilled manual employee Machine operator	1	0.5
Semiskilled employee	0	0.0
Unskilled employee Unemployed	3	1.6

III. Fathers of Down Syndrome Population

Age distribution (years): Range: (20–50)
Mean: 32.27
Median: 30
STD dev.: 6.23

Race:

	N	%
None given	2	1.1
Caucasian	147	77.4
Black	4	2.1
Hispanic	32	16.8
Jewish	4	2.1
Other	1	0.5

Religion:

	N	%
No data	64	33.7
None	21	11.1
Catholic	50	26.3
Protestant	30	15.8
Jewish	9	4.7
Other	16	8.4

Father's education:

Years	N	%
No information	15	7.9
4	1	0.5
7	1	0.5
9	1	0.5
10	2	1.1
11	5	2.6
12	45	23.7
13	9	4.7
14	22	11.6
15	8	4.2
16	41	21.6
17	5	2.6
18	22	11.6

	N	%
19	5	2.6
20	5	2.6
21	1	0.5
22	2	1.1

Mean: 14.73 STD dev. 4.80

Father living in home (intact family):

	N	%
No data	8	4.2
Yes	169	88.9
No	13	6.8

Father's occupation:

	N	%
No information	27	14.2
Owner of large firm Higher executive Major professional	29	15.3
Business manager Owner of medium business Lesser professional	32	16.8
Owner of small independent business Administrative personnel Minor professional	34	17.9
Technician/clerical/sales person Owner of very small business	22	11.6
Skilled/manual employee Machine operator	33	17.4
Semiskilled employee	8	4.2
Unskilled employee Unemployed	5	2.6

2. Comparison of Gross Motor Developmental Milestone Attainment

	Children with Down Syndrome		Other Children	
Activity	Age in Months	Range	Age in Months	Range
Hold head steady & balanced	5	3–9	3	1–4
Rolls over	8	4–12	5	1–4
Sits without support for one minute or more	9	6–16	7	5–9
Pulls to stand using furniture	15	8–26	8	7–12
Walks with support	16	6–30	10	7–12
Stands alone	18	12–38	11	9–16
Walks alone	19	13–48	12	9–17
Walks up stairs with help	30	20–48	17	12–24
Walks down stairs with help	36	24–60+	17	13–24

Source: Adapted from Cunningham, C. (1982). *Down syndrome: An introduction for parents*. London: Souvenir Press.

3. Comparison of Fine Motor and Adaptive Milestone Attainment

	Children with Down Syndrome		Other Children	
Activity	Age in Months	Range	Age in Months	Range
Follows objects with eyes	3	1–6	1	1–3
Grasps dangling ring	6	4–11	4	2–6
Transfers	8	6–12	5	4–8
Pulls string to attain toy	11	7–17	7	5–10
Uncovers toy	13	9–21	8	6–12
Places objects into cup	19	12–34	12	9–18
Builds tower of two cubes	20	14–32	14	10–19
Completes simple three-shape jigsaw	33	20–48	22	16–30
Copies a circle	48	36–60	30	24–40
Matches shapes and colors	4–5 yrs.			

Source: Adapted from Cunningham, C. (1982). *Down syndrome: An introduction for parents*. London: Souvenir Press.

4. Cardiac Conditions

Cardiac problems of children who participated in a study conducted at the City of Hope National Medical Center, Duarte, California.

1. Functional murmur.
2. Flow murmur.
3. Heart murmur.
4. Functional murmur, rule out atrial septal defect.
5. Irregular heart rate.
6. Heart murmur, small ventricular septal defect.
7. Heart murmur, rule out atrial septal defect.
8. Heart murmur, rule out ventricular septal defect.
9. Heart murmur, rule out ventricular septal defect or endocardial cushion.
10. Mitral valve prolapse.
11. Pulmonary valve stenosis.
12. Aortic stenosis.
13. Patent ductus arteriosus.
14. Patent ductus arteriosus (small).
15. Ventricular septal defect.
16. Ventricular septal defect (closed).
17. Ventricular septal defect (status post repair).
18. Ventricular septal defect/pulmonary stenosis.
19. Atrial venous canal.
20. Atrial septal defect/venous canal.
21. Endocardial cushion.
22. Atrial venous canal (status post correction).
23. Atrial venous canal/deformed mitral valve.
24. Atrial venous canal/mitral regurgitation.
25. Atrial septal defect.
26. Atrial septal defect/ventricular septal defect.
27. Atrial venous canal/mitral regurgitation pulmonary hypertension.
28. Atrial venous canal/patent ductus arteriosus.
29. Patent ductus arteriosus/atrial septal defect.
30. Ventricular septal defect/patent ductus arteriosus/atrial septal defect.
31. Ventricular septal defect/patent ductus arteriosus/atrial septal defect/mitral insufficiency.
32. Absent mitral valve aortic stenosis/ventricular septal defect.
33. Ventricular septal defect/patent ductus arteriosus/atrial septal defect/pulmonary hypertension.
34. Tetralogy of fallot.

5. Summary of the Results of the Sample's Performance on the Bayley Scales of Infant Development by Age

		Mental			Psychomotor		
Subject	Chronological age in months	Raw score	Index score	Developmental age in months	Raw score	Index score	Developmental age in months
1	02	10	64	1	10	93	2
2	02	18	80	1	m[a]	m	m
3	02	27	94	2	m	m	m
4	02	25	100	2	10	93	2
5	03	15	63	1	13	88	3
6	03	28	75	2	11	75	2
7	03	29	77	2	9	75	2
8	03	35	86	3	13	84	3
9	04	36	88	3	m	m	m
10	04	15	38	1	7	54	1
11	04	26	54	2	12	67	2
12	05	46	89	4	11	62	2
13	05	48	94	4	m	m	m
14	05	63	106	5	18	78	4
15	05	53	79	5	16	69	4
16	06	46	61	4	16	63	4
17	06	52	68	5	23	66	5
18	06	46	61	4	49	74	5
19	06	77	110	7	m	m	m
20	07	74	86	6	27	80	6
21	07	75	88	6	24	73	6
22	07	62	63	5	27	84	6
23	08	73	68	6	23	54	5
24	08	67	66	6	24	57	6
25	08	83	98	8	25	60	6
26	08	75	73	6	17	> .3[b]	4
27	09	76	67	6	24	> .3	6
28	09	79	74	7	33	76	7
29	09	74	63	6	33	76	7
30	09	82	83	8	32	72	7
31	10	80	67	7	29	50	6
32	10	87	84	9	36	72	8
33	10	82	72	8	27	> .3	6
34	10	87	84	9	31	57	7
35	11	83	62	8	35	61	8
36	11	90	79	9	31	> .3	7
37	11	90	79	9	35	61	8
38	11	93	88	10	38	69	9
39	12	87	58	9	36	55	8
40	12	83	50	8	31	> .3	7
41	13	91	62	10	34	> .3	8
42	13	95	72	10	40	62	9
43	14	94	61	10	39	55	9
44	14	98	70	11	42	67	10
45	14	94	61	10	33	> .3	7
46	14	99	72	11	m	m	m
47	15	93	50	10	36	> .3	9
48	15	104	75	12	38	> .3	9

Table 5. (*Cont.*)

Subject	Chronological age in months	Mental: Raw score	Mental: Index score	Mental: Developmental age in months	Psychomotor: Raw score	Psychomotor: Index score	Psychomotor: Developmental age in months
49	15	93	50	10	40	54	9
50	16	98	54	11	44	11	11
51	17	113	78	15	48	78	14
52	17	108	67	14	m	m	m
53	17	87	>.3	9	40	50	9
54	18	92	>.3	10	43	57	11
55	19	99	>.3	11	m	m	m
56	19	m	m	m	43	50	11
57	21	118	62	16	m	m	m
58	21	106	>.3	13	48	54	14
59	21	119	64	16	48	54	14
60	21	90	>.3	9	36	>.3	8
61	22	125	74	18	m	m	m
62	22	124	72	18	55	84	18
63	22	108	>.3	14	48	53	14
64	22	126	76	18	51	63	16
65	22	m	m	m	43	>.3	11
66	22	122	68	17	44	>.3	11
67	23	117	56	16	48	50	14
68	26	125	61	18	44	>.3	11
69	28	118	>.3	16	m	m	m
70	28	135	67	21	53	58	17
71	28	129	59	19	55	65	18
72	28	119	>.3	16	54	61	17
73	29	137	67	21	m	m	m
74	29	133	61	20	54	61	17
75	29	118	>.3	16	48	>.3	14
76	30	63	>.3	5	22	>.3	5
77	30	84	>.3	8	40	>.3	9
78	30	149	>.3	25	52	>.3	16

[a]m represents children not tested for that scale.
[b]>.3 represents greater than minus three standard deviations below the mean.

6. Summary of Schnell (1984) Results

Mean raw scores and developmental age for a longitudinal sample of children with Down syndrome on the Bayley scales of Infant Development.

Mental Development			
Age in months	N	Raw scores	Developmental ages
6	81	39.8	3.3
12	88	73.9	6.7
18	75	94.6	10.5
24	80	108.2	13.6
30	80	119.6	16.7
36	75	133.0	20.6
Psychomotor Development			
Age in months	N	Raw scores	Developmental ages
6	81	17.2	4.0
12	83	31.9	7.2
18	75	41.8	10.4
24	80	46.9	13.1
30	80	52.0	16.6
36	75	55.2	19.0

Source: Schnell R.R. (1984). Psychomotor development. In S.Pueschel (Ed.), *The young child with Down syndrome* (p. 212). New York: Sciences Press.

7. Distribution of the Sample of Children with Down Syndrome on the Bayley Scales of Infant Development

	Total sample	Mental scale sample	Psychomotor scale sample
	n	n	n
Mental scale only	12	12	0
Psychomotor scale only	2	0	2
Both scales	64	64	64
Total sample	78	76	66

8. Summary of the Raw Scores and Developmental Ages on the Mental Scale of the Bayley Scales of Infant Development of Children with Down Syndrome (N = 76)

Age groups in months	N=	Raw score Mean	Raw score SD	Developmental ages Mean	Developmental ages SD
2	4	20	7.7	1.5	0.6
3	4	26.7	8.4	2.0	0.8
4	3	25.6	10.5	2.0	1.0
5	4	52.5	7.6	4.5	0.6
6	4	55.2	14.8	5.0	1.4
7–8	7	72.7	6.7	6.1	0.9
9–10	8	80.9	4.7	7.5	1.2
11–12	6	87.7	4.1	8.8	0.8
13–15	9	95.6	4.0	10.4	0.7
16–18	5	99.6	10.8	11.8	2.6
19–21	5	106.4	12.4	13.0	3.0
22–24	6	120.3	6.8	14.3	6.7
25–27	1	125.0	0.0	18.0	0.0
28–30	10	118.5	26.1	16.7	6.1

9. Summary of the Raw Scores and Developmental Ages on the Psychomotor Scale of the Bayley Scales of Infant Development of Children with Down Syndrome (N = 66)

Age groups in months	N=	Raw score Mean	Raw score SD	Developmental ages Mean	Developmental ages SD
2	2	10.0	0.0	1.5	0.7
3	4	11.5	1.9	2.2	0.5
4	2	9.5	3.5	1.5	0.7
5	3	15.0	3.6	3.7	1.5
6	3	19.3	3.5	4.7	0.6
7–8	7	23.8	3.4	5.4	0.5
9–10	8	30.6	3.8	6.7	0.7
11–12	6	34.3	2.8	7.8	0.8
13–15	8	37.7	3.1	8.7	0.9
16–18	4	43.7	3.3	11.2	2.1
19–21	4	43.7	5.7	11.7	2.9
22–24	6	48.2	4.4	14.0	2.7
25–27	1	44.0	0.0	11.0	0.0
28–30	8	47.2	11.3	14.1	4.7

10.1. Standardized Anthropometric Techniques

All measurements were taken on the left side of the body by two nutritionists trained in the use of standardized anthropometric techniques. Duplicate measures were taken and repeated if not within accepted tolerance limits. The average of the duplicate measures was used. If the second set of measurements was not acceptable, the mean of all four measurements was used. The equipment was maintained regularly to ensure accuracy. A standard 600-mm rod was used to check the stadiometer, standard weights were used to calibrate the scale, and a calibration block was used to verify the accuracy of the calipers.

Weight. Children wearing underpants only were weighed on a balance-beam scale. Infants were undressed completely and weighed on an infant scale. Readings were made to the nearest 0.1 kg. Accepted tolerance limit was 0.1 kg. If the child refused to stand, sit, or lie on the scale, the parent was weighed first, and then reweighed holding the child. The difference between weights was taken as the weight of the child.

Height/Length. Stature was measured on all children over 3 years of age using a Harpenden stadiometer. Measurements were taken with the heels, buttocks, shoulder blades, and back of the head touching the vertical plane. Overweight children, whose body contour did not permit that position, stood slightly away from that plane, but with the buttocks still in contact. Measurements were made to the nearest 0.1 cm. Accepted tolerance limit was 1.0 cm.

Infant length was measured using an infant board constructed according to a standard model. Measurements were made to the nearest 0.1 cm, with one nutritionist holding the child's crown against the stationary headboard while the other positioned the child's thighs and adjusted the footboard so it was firmly placed against the soles of the child's feet. Accepted tolerance limit was 1.0 cm.

Sitting Height/Crown-Rump. Sitting height in children over 3 years of age was measured using the stadiometer and a special box constructed to be exactly 50 cm high. The child was seated on the box and the same procedure was followed as for height measurement. Sitting height was calculated by subtracting 50 cm from the resulting figure. Accepted tolerance limit was 1.0 cm.

Infant crown-rump length was measured using the length board. The child's legs were bent so the things were perpendicular to the board and the foot board pressed firmly against the buttocks. Accepted tolerance limit was 0.5 cm.

Arm/Head Circumferences. Arm and head circumferences were measured using an insertion tape. The largest circumference of the occiput of the head was obtained while maintaining the tape in a stationary position just above the eyebrow (supraorbital ridge). Measurements were recorded to the nearest 0.1 cm. Accepted tolerance limit was 0.2 cm.

Arm circumference was measured at the midpoint between the olecranon and acromion processes (determined with the arm flexed at 90 deg), with the arm dangling and relaxed. Measurements were recorded to the nearest 0.1 cm. Accepted tolerance limit was 0.2 cm.

Skinfolds. Skinfold measurements were taken using Lange calipers at the triceps site, midway between the olecranon and acromion processes with the arm dangling and relaxed. The reading was made after 3 seconds to the nearest 0.5 mm. Accepted tolerance limit was 3.0 cm. The subscapular skinfold was measured, using the same technique, below the tip of the scapula at a 45 degree angle to the spine.

10.2. Recommendations for Nutrition Assessment of the Child with Down Syndrome

Anthropometry

Stature. Because of the short stature and abnormal growth pattern in children with Down syndrome, it is preferable to use the growth grids developed specifically for this disorder (see Figures 10.1–10.4) to evaluate the child's stature. As with normal children, it is better to plot serial measurements in order to determine if the child's growth *rate* has been normal, especially if he/she presently appears to be of short stature (< 10th percentile). Unless the child has severe heart disease, there appears to be no need to alter the assessment protocol.

Weight. Weight should also be evaluated using the Down syndrome specific growth grids when possible. The child's weight should be at approximately the same percentile as his/her height. Weight for stature can be compared to the NCHS reference data, since those are age-independent.

Skinfold Measurements. In order to evaluate whether a child who appears to be overweight is really overfat, skinfold measurements should be made in conjunction with weight measurements. Our preliminary analyses suggest that using the NCHS reference data is appropriate for triceps skinfold measurements. However, these analyses also suggest that the subscapular skinfold measurements of our study population do not "fit" those of the normal reference population, either NCHS (Johnson) or Fomon. Further analyses/studies are needed to determine whether these children have a different body-fat distribution.

Midarm/Arm-Muscle circumferences. The midarm circumference, in conjunction with the triceps skinfold measurement, allows one to calculate the arm muscle circumference and/or area. This provides additional information regarding the child's body composition. Since our preliminary analyses suggest that children with Down syndrome may have increased muscle mass it may be important to also use this information to evaluate whether an overweight child is really overfat or obese.

Head Circumference. Since children with Down syndrome are significantly microcephalic when compared to normal reference data, and no Down syndrome-specific reference data exist, a single measurement is not of much use. However, in children 3 years and under, it is still important to monitor the growth of the head to detect any abnormalities (e.g., flattening of the curve) in a timely fashion, although the reasons for these abnormalities are often not related to the child's nutritional status.

Dietary

Energy. Energy needs should be assessed based on height as well as age. Assessment of the adequacy of energy intake should take into consideration both dietary and anthropometric data, and be reevaluated periodically in relation to individual weight gain and estimated body composition using skinfold data.

Nutrients. Micronutrient needs (vitamins and minerals) should probably also be assessed taking size into consideration as well as age, especially since the RDA for some nutrients (e.g., thiamin, riboflavin) is based on energy intake. Special attention should be paid to the dietary sources of those nutrients for which children with Down syndrome may be at risk: vitamin A, pyridoxine, and zinc. At the same time, it should be ascertained whether caregivers are giving children unprescribed supplements at levels that may be toxic.

Biochemical

Routine biochemical tests are not recommended unless dietary and clinical assessments indicate suspected energy/nutrient deficiencies. Clinical indications might include frequent infections, which, coupled with a low dietary intake of vitamin A or zinc, might warrant biochemical investigation of the child's vitamin A and/or zinc status.

If a child is being supplemented with "megadoses" of vitamins, it is important to determine if the supplement is providing nutrients at potentially toxic levels. However, although the clinician has an obligation to protect the child from harmful substances and must share scientific knowledge with caregivers, we may lose credibility with those caregivers by totally dismissing such controversial therapies, especially if the caregivers believe they make a difference to the child's well-being.

Feeding

If nutrition screening indicates a delay in feeding skill development or that the child is eating foods inappropriate for his/her developmental level, a feeding assessment should be considered. This assessment will ideally include an oral pharyngeal/neuromuscular assessment and a behavioral assessment to complement the nutrition evaluation (Ogg, 1975).

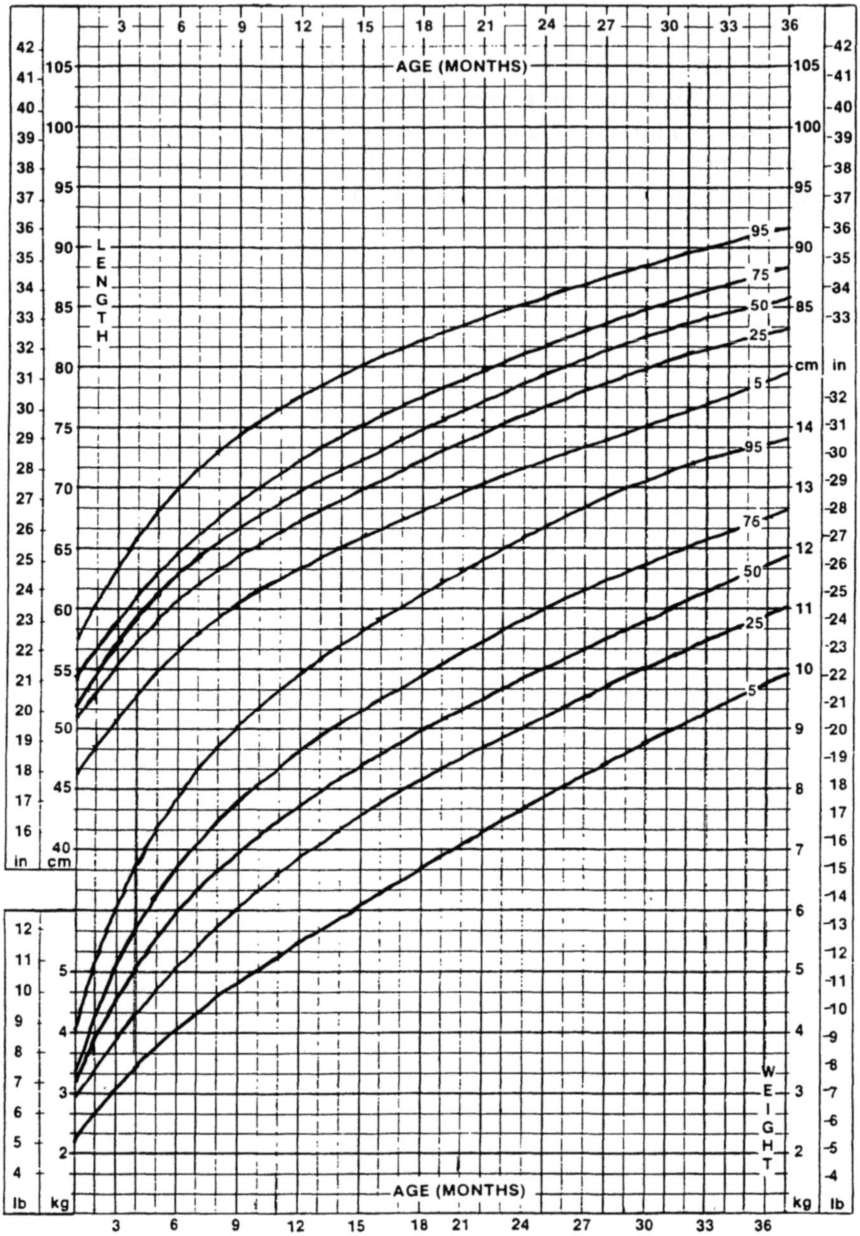

FIGURE 10.1. Height and weight for females with Down syndrome, birth to 36 months of age, based on mixed longitudinal data on approximately 300 girls with Down syndrome born between 1960 and 1986 and reared at home. Children with congenital heart disease are included in the sample. Data collected at the Developmental Evaluation Clinic of the Children's Hospital Boston, The Child Development Center of Rhode Island Hospital, and the Clinical Genetics Service of the Children's Hospital of Philadelphia.
Source: Copyright, Cronk, C.E. et al.: Pediatrics 81:102, 1988.

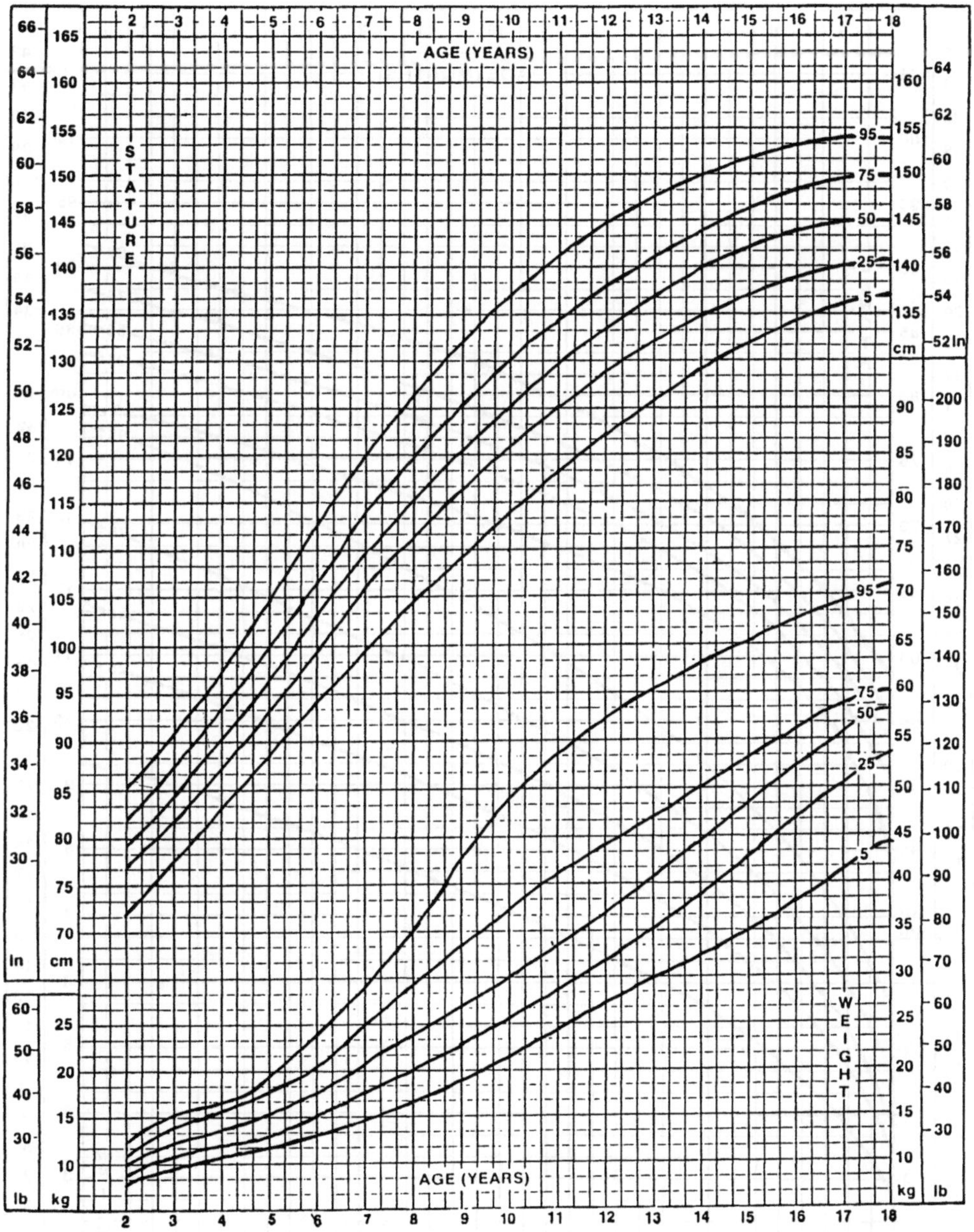

FIGURE 10.2. Height and weight for females with Down syndrome 2 to 18 years of age based on mixed longitudinal data on approximately 300 girls with Down syndrome born between 1960 and 1986 and reared at home. Children with congenital heart disease are included in the sample. See Figure 10.1 for further details.
Source: Cronk, C.E. et al.: Pediatrics 81:102, 1988.

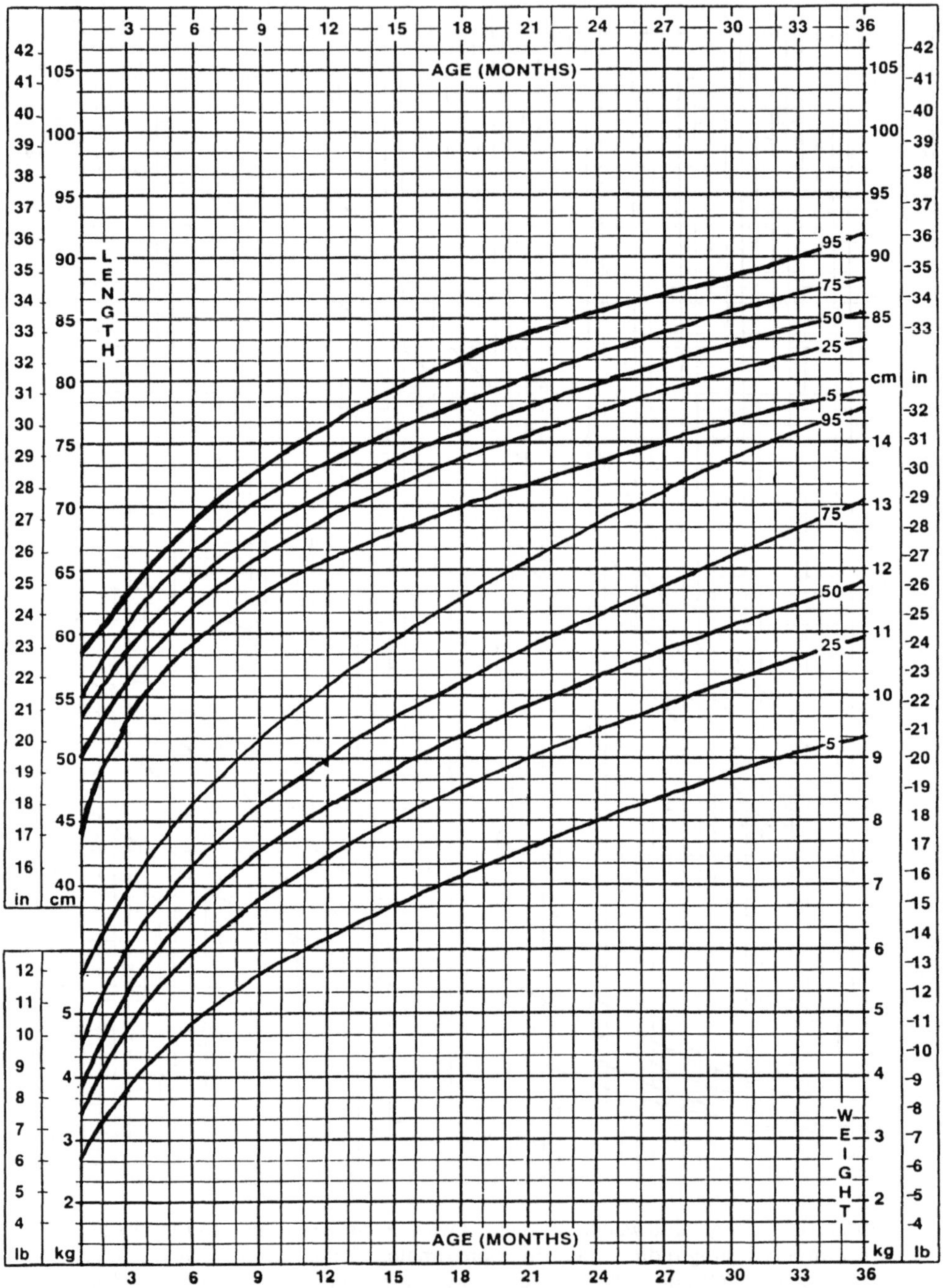

FIGURE 10.3. Height and weight for males with Down syndrome birth to 36 months of age based on mixed longitudinal data for approximately 400 boys with Down syndrome born between 1960 and 1986 and reared at home. Children with congenital heart disease are included in the sample. See Figure 10.1 for further details. *Source:* Cronk, C.E. et al.: Pediatrics 81:102, 1988.

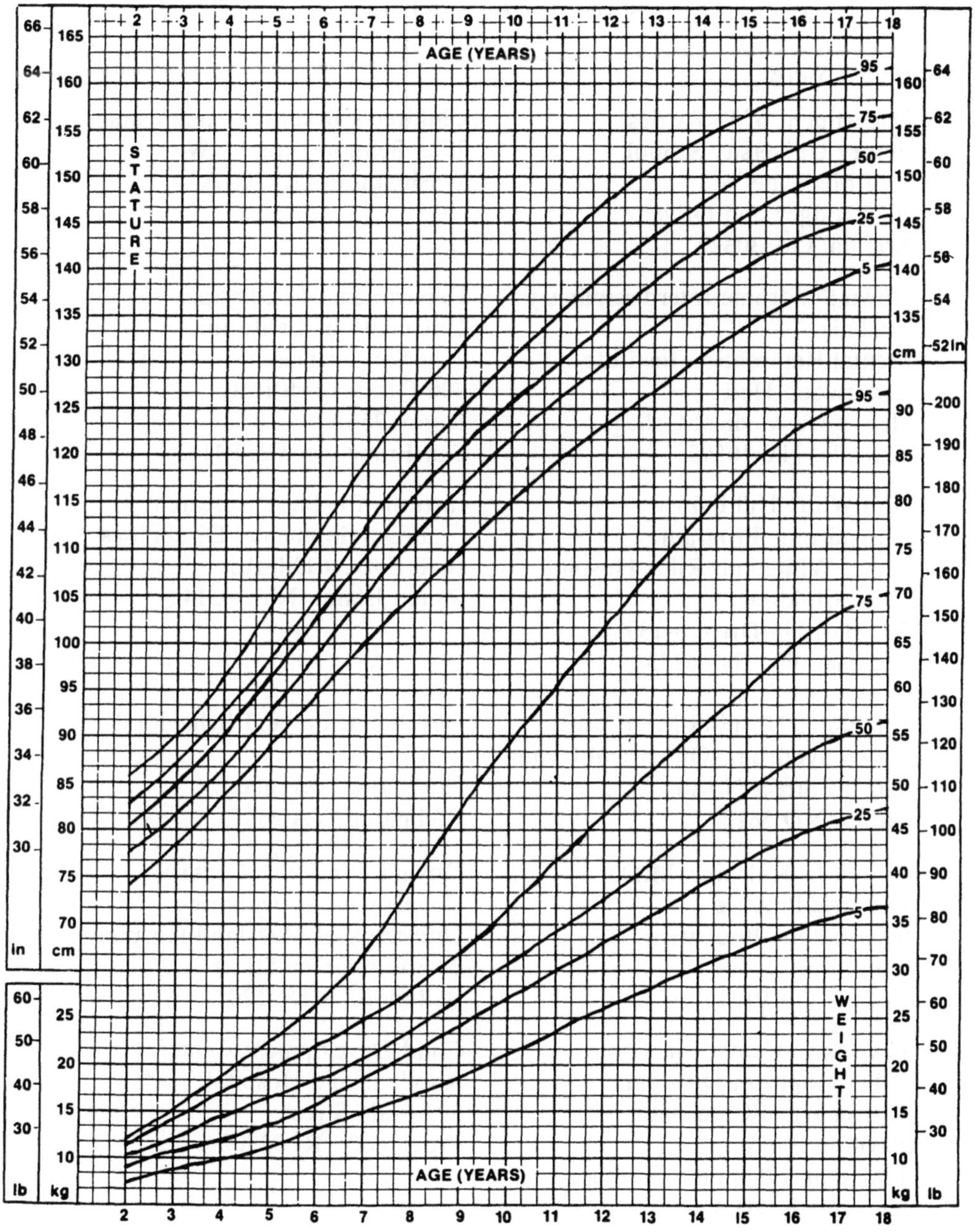

FIGURE 10.4. Height and weight for males with Down syndrome 2 to 18 years of age based on mixed longitudinal data for approximately 400 boys with Down syndrome born between 1960 and 1984 and reared at home. Children with congenital heart disease are included in the sample. See Figure 10.1 for further details.
Source: Cronk, et al.: Pediatrics 81:102, 1988.

11. Medical Clinics for Down Syndrome

United States

Department of Pediatrics
Emory University School
of Medicine
2040 Ridgewood Drive
Atlanta, GA 30322

Down Syndrome Interdisciplinary
Clinic
Mental Retardation Institute
Cedarwood Hall
New York Medical College
Valhalla, NY 10595

Ann White Hill Down
Syndrome Program
James Whitcomb Riley Hospital
for Children
702 Barnhill Drive S-139
Indianapolis, IN 46223

Children's Hospital-Merit Care
Down Syndrome Outpatient Clinic
720 4th Street North
Fargo, ND 58122

Milton L. Kolchins, M.D.
Pediatric Practice
5400 Balboa Boulevard
Suite 105
Encino, CA 91316

Cincinnati Center for
Development Disorders
University of Cincinnati
Pavilion Building
Elland and Bethesda Avenues
Cincinnati, OH 45229

La Rabida Children's Hospital
and Research Center
East 65th Street at Lake Michigan
Chicago, IL 60649

Children's Brain Research Clinic
2525 Belmont Road NW
Washington, DC 20008

Department of Pediatrics
University of California
at San Francisco
400 Parnassus Street
Room 266A
San Francisco, CA 94143

Institute for Basic Research
in Developmental Disabilities
1050 Forrest Hill Rd.
Staten Island, NY 10314

Developmental and Behavioral
Medicine
7834 Forest Avenue
Richmond, VA 23225

Down's Syndrome Center
Department of Pediatrics
University of Maryland Hospital
22 South Green Street
Baltimore, MD 21201

Child Development Center
Rhode Island Hospital
593 Eddy Street
Providence, RI 02902

Blick Clinic for Developmental
Disabilities
640 West Market Street
Akron, OH 44303

Down Syndrome Program
The Children's Hospital—Boston
300 Longwood Avenue
Boston, MA 02115

The Bancroft School
Hopkins Lane
Haddonfield, NJ 08033

Children's Hospital Medical Center
of Northern California
51st and Grove Street
Oakland, CA 94609

Regional Genetic Consultative Clinic
The University of Iowa
Hospitals and Clinics
Iowa City, IA 52242

Down Syndrome Clinic
Department of Pediatrics
Medical College of Ohio
300 Arlington Avenue
Toledo, OH 43699

Santa Rosa Birth Defects Center
University of Texas Health
Science Center
P.O. Box 7330 Station A
San Antonio, TX 78285

Outside the United States

Fundacion Sindrone de Down
de Canabria
Universidad de Santander
Santander, Spain

Center Medic Down
Valencia 231
4°4°a 08007
Barcelona, Spain

Yamanashi Medical College
Department of Health Science
Tamaho, Nakakomo
Yamanashi, 409-38 Japan

St. Vincenz Krankenhaus
Am Busdorf 4 A
4790 Paderborn
Federal Republic of Germany

Wildbohn 45
Frankfurt Oder
German Democratic Republic 1201

Centre Surrey
University of Toronto
2 Surrey Place
Toronto, Ontario
Canada
M5S-2C2

Institute de Progenese
45 rue des Saint Peres
75270
Paris Cedex 06
France

12. Computerized Assessment Forms

- Demographic data form.
- History form.
- Physical assessment form.
- Laboratory data form.
- Dental assessment form.
- ENT assessment form.
- Audiology assessment form.
- Audiology questionnaire.
- Physical therapy assessment form.
- Occupational therapy assessment form.
- Psychology assessment form.
- Summary nutritional report.
- Measurement form.
- Nutritional questionnaire.

All forms are available from:
Don C. Van Dyke, M.D.
University Hospital School
The University of Iowa
Iowa City, IA 52242

13. Ten Commandments[1]

1. Take one day at a time, and take that day positively. You do not have control over the future, but you do have control over today.
2. Never underestimate your child's potential. Allow him or her, encourage him or her, expect him or her to develop to the best of his abilities.
3. Find and follow positive mentors: parents and professionals who can share their experience, advice, and support.
4. Provide and be involved with the most appropriate educational and learning environments for your child from infancy on.
5. Keep in mind the feelings and needs of your spouse and your other children. Remind them that this child does not get more of your love just because he or she may get more of your time.
6. Answer only to your conscience; then you will be able to answer to your child. You need not justify your actions to your friends or the public.
7. Be honest with your feelings. You cannot be a super-parent 24 hours a day. Allow yourself jealousy, anger, pity, frustration, and depression in small amounts whenever necessary.
8. Be kind to yourself. Do not focus continually on what needs to be done. Remember to look at what you have accomplished.
9. Stop and smell the roses. Take advantage of the fact that you have gained a special appreciation for the little miracles in life that others take for granted.
10. Keep and use a sense of humor. Cracking up with laughter can keep you from cracking up with stress.

[1]O'Halloran, J. *Down syndrome Congress newsletter*, Sept. 1986.

Index

MIX
Papier aus verantwortungsvollen Quellen
Paper from responsible sources
FSC® C105338
FSC
www.fsc.org

If you have any concerns about our products,
you can contact us on
ProductSafety@springernature.com

In case Publisher is established outside the EU,
the EU authorized representative is:
Springer Nature Customer Service Center GmbH
Europaplatz 3, 69115 Heidelberg, Germany

Printed by Libri Plureos GmbH
in Hamburg, Germany